Florence Nightingale and the Water Cure

by

Cora Weaver

To my dearest friend Wendy
from Cora

Published by
CORA WEAVER
Malvern

Cora Weaver, 4 Hall Green, Malvern, Worcestershire WR14 3QX

The front cover picture is a photograph of Florence Nightingale c.1853-4 when she was Superintendent of the Upper Harley Street Establishment for Gentlewomen.
Photograph courtesy of Florence Nightingale Museum Trust, London.

ISBN 978-1-873809-87-7

Contents

Notes in [ ] are author's comments

Illustrations

Dramatis Personae

Florence Nightingale (1820-1910)
W.E.N - William Edward Nightingale, né Shore (1794-1874), Florence's father
Fanny - Fanny Nightingale, née Smith (1788-1880), Florence's mother
Parthe - Frances Parthenope Nightingale (1819-1890), Florence's sister, later Lady Verney
Aunt Mai (1798-1889), Mary Shore, W.E.N's sister, married Fanny's brother Samuel Smith
Aunt Julia (1799-1883), Julia Smith, Fanny's sister
Hilary Bonham Carter (1821-1865), Florence's cousin; daughter of Fanny's sister Joanna
Arthur Clough (1819-1861), married to Aunt Mai's daughter
Blanche William Shore Smith (1831-1894), Aunt Mai's son,
Florence's cousin

The Author

Cora Florence Weaver, M.St (*Oxon*), has lived in Malvern, Worcestershire, for thirty two years and has written and published works on various aspects of the county's history. Her particular interests lie in the origins and development of English spas, particularly Malvern and Droitwich, and in the Worcestershire life of Sir Edward Elgar, areas on which she writes, publishes, lectures and broadcasts.

She became interested in the life and work of Florence Nightingale when she started teaching the subject to Year 2 children in schools throughout Worcestershire and in the Midlands. Following a visit to the Florence Nightingale museum at the former Barrack Hospital at Scutari, and visits to Claydon House and the Florence Nightingale Museum in London, Cora set out to discover more about Florence Nightingale's visits to Malvern.

Acknowledgements

I most gratefully acknowledge the following institutions and individuals for their collective help in making this book possible.

To Sir Edmund Verney of Claydon House, for making available the archive of Nightingale family letters; to Sue Baxter (Archivist), Claydon House Trust, for her invaluable and capacious advice and help in a variety of matters; to Kirsteen Nixon, Collections Manager at the Florence Nightingale Museum, London, for her assistance in the loan of images from the Florence Nightingale Museum Trust's collection; to the Wellcome Library, a resource open to everybody, for allowing the unlimited use of its extensive archive and the amusing and friendly support I received from one particular librarian; to the Henry Bonham Carter Will Trust for allowing the unlimited use of quotations from the Nightingale family letters; to the British Library for assistance in locating relevant letters in its collection; to Roger Hall Jones for the loan of an unusual cartoon image of the water cure; to Dr Bruce Osborne of the Spas Research Fellowship for access to the SRF archives; to Brian Iles and Chris and Roland Bannister for access to their archives of historic images; to John Fenwick of Umberslade Hall for kindly allowing access to the private building and its grounds; to Malcolm Neesam for identifying Mrs Wright's lodging house in Harrogate. Finally, I am indebted to previously published works on the life and work of Florence Nightingale, notably *Florence Nightingale* by Cecil Woodham Smith; *Florence Nightingale, The Woman and her Legend* by Mark Bostridge, and the mammoth 'Collected Works of Florence Nightingale' edited by Lynn McDonald.

This book is dedicated to my mother, Florence.

Introduction

Benjamin Jowett wrote to Florence Nightingale from West Malvern on 31st December 1879. He told her that there had been such a great deal of romantic feeling about her 23 years earlier, when she came home from the Crimea, that she might have become a duchess if she had played her cards right. He said that because of her, thousands of girls aged between 18 and 23 were named Florence; that she was a myth in her own life time. Now, he said, she had disappeared from public view, working in silence so that her nurses might save lives in hospitals. Since she had introduced a new era in nursing, many thousand of soldiers were no longer the victims of bad water, bad drainage, bad air and bad ventilation. Hundreds of thousands of native Indians, in this generation and in generations to come, had been saved 'by the energy of a sick lady who can scarcely rise from her bed'. The world , he said, neither knew of these things nor thought of them.

The life and work of this myth in her own lifetime, this 'sick lady' has been examined and interpreted many times since her death on 13th August 1910. She is perhaps the world's most famous invalid, renowned for taking to her bed for almost half her life. Different writers have attributed different reasons for this prolonged confinement. Some suggest that it may have been the result of the horrors at Scutari and in the Crimea, compounded with the stress of pushing through the inquiry into the health of the army; or it may have been the result of family difficulties with her demanding mother and sister. Other writers have flung accusations of malingering, or of feigning illness, suggesting that this was unnecessary and unacceptable behaviour.

This book examines her illness and how she tried to resolve it.

Chapter I
Doctors, Medicine & Hospitals versus The Water Cure

Florence Nightingale habitually avoided her own incarceration in hospitals when she was unwell. In general she had no time for doctors, for drugs, or for hospitals. Of the first she wrote, 'I have no faith in medicine... As people put in the "Marriages" the name of the clergyman... who married them, I would put in the "Deaths" the name of the doctor or doctors who had killed them.' Of the second she commented that medicine could not cure; only Nature could cure. Of the third she wrote in a report of 1853 that hospitals were only useful for the seriously ill. She said that prolonged incarceration by the moderately ill turned hospitals into lodging houses where nervous, foolish, idle and selfish people became even more nervous, foolish, idle and selfish, and homeless patients invented complaints as a means of extending their stay. Generally, only workhouse hospitals admitted and maintained the chronic sick so at the Gentlewomen's hospital in Upper Harley Street, where she worked as superintendent in 1853, her patients were discharged after two months.

The extended Nightingale family and their friends were much in favour of taking the Water Cure - which Florence Nightingale considered a Nature cure - for a variety of complaints, in spas at home and abroad. Perhaps the earliest reference to this is in a letter of 6th September 1828, when Florence was eight years old, and prone to illnesses and weakness of the hands and ankles. Her great aunt, Maria Coape, wrote to Flo's mother, 'I suppose you find it really necessary for Night. and Flo to take the Cheltenham waters...' The resort to spas for curative purposes will raise eyebrows in Britain where, with a few exceptions, we have lost the knowledge and understanding of the benefits of spa treatment in regaining health, and our physicians no longer have the skills to implement such treatment, as they do in most other European countries.

John and Mrs Smedley practised hydropathy at Matlock

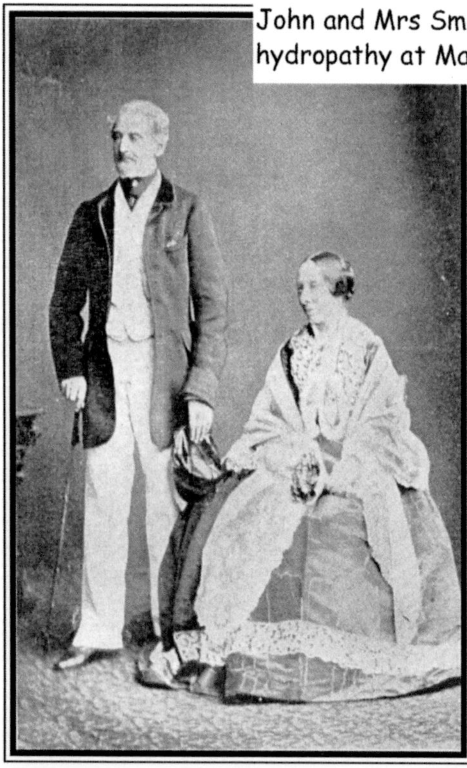

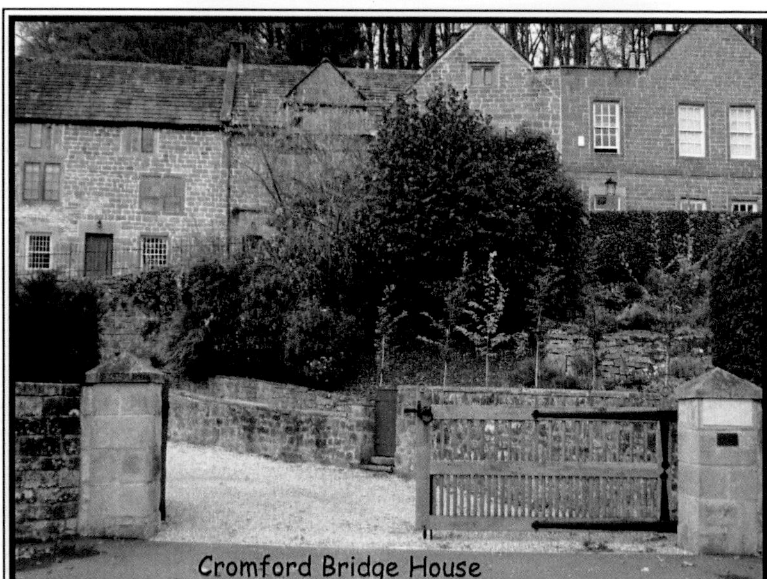

Cromford Bridge House

Florence Nightingale on the Water Cure

Florence Nightingale spent many of her early summers at the family's northern home of Lea Hurst, a short distance from the popular spa town of Matlock, where John Smedley (1801-75), with the assistance of his wife, ran a vast and successful hydropathic establishment. The Nightingales and the Smedleys were old allies. In 1784 John's father and W.E.N's uncle, Peter Nightingale, had established a muslin and cotton spinning empire based at Lea Mills, near Lea Hurst. By 1818 the Smedleys were living at Cromford Bridge House, near Lea Hurst and for several years young John Smedley was one of Florence's neighbours. When the Smedleys left Cromford Bridge House it became the home of Florence's great aunt, Elizabeth Evans. When she died in 1852, Fanny offered the house to her younger daughter to run as a small hospital. Flo was pleased with the recognition of her aims but declined the offer, as she did not feel ready to take on such a challenge.

The Nightingale family letters are sprinkled with examples of people they knew who went to Matlock for treatment. Over the years Florence learned that, if incorrectly prescribed, hydropathy could be a water-kill rather than a water-cure. She would not trust any woman, including herself, to say whether someone either needed, or could benefit from, the cold water cure: that, she said, should only be done by a doctor and the treatment should and always, and only, be taken under a doctor's instructions. Unfortunately good hydropathic doctors were rare. In 1860 she knew of only one in London who could give an impartial opinion as to whether a patient needed the Water Cure,* and outside the capital there was really only Dr Gully in Malvern. However he had such a large and prosperous practice that he would disappear for weeks and leave his patients to a third-rate practitioner, to the detriment of the patients.

Florence believed that the term 'hydropathic treatment' misled people into believing that ailments could be cured by the use of water

* Sir James Clark (1788-1870), Queen Victoria's medical adviser. It was with his support that Florence secured the superintendency at the Harley Street hospital.

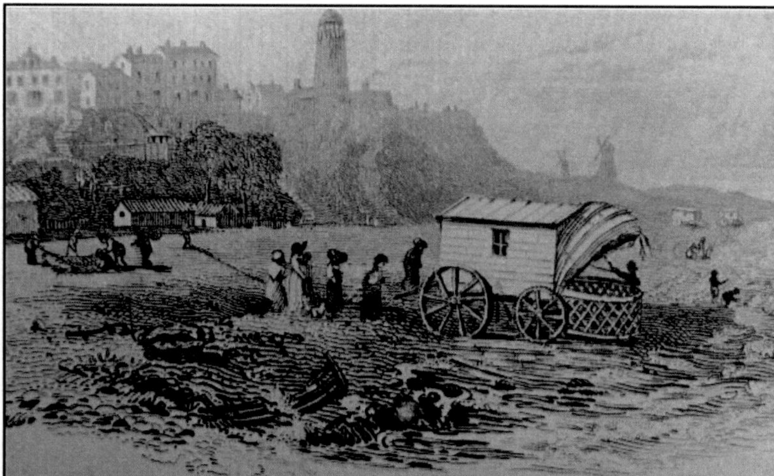

Florence and Hilary doused in from the top step of a bathing machine.

alone. Water, she wrote, was just one element of a package that included absence from a stressful environment (such as Parliament), 'absence from head excitement, absence from night hours, proper diet, quiet life, exercise, fresh mountain air, and different kinds of bathing'. She added that when water was used on its own it 'has not achieved cure – shewing that it is the whole way of life, not the particular specific which brings about the cure.' She described it as being more of a nature treatment than a water treatment; and it is one that is largely recommended in the twenty-first century for the regaining and maintenance of good health.

Florence Nightingale and Sea Bathing

In October 1833 Fanny Nightingale and her sister Julia took three young teenagers - Florence, Parthenope and their cousin Hilary Bonham Carter - and Hilary's eight-year-old brother Alfred, for a month's healthy holiday to Seaview, a suburb of Ryde on the Isle of Wight. Fanny returned home on the 16th, leaving Aunt Julia in charge. The holiday was a mixture of drawing and bible reading every morning, as Fanny had instructed, often visiting friends and relatives on the mainland, walking along the sand to places of interest, collecting shells, and bathing. Florence described to her mother how on the 17th she and Hilary had a tepid bath at the baths and two days later took their first dip in the sea. They stood holding hands on the top step of a bathing machine then 'doused in' three times. 'The first dip was wretched cold, but afterwards I got warm and enjoyed the second and third dips very much. I have got no cold, and I think it has made me warm for the whole day.'

They dived for white pebbles in the sea, walked along the pier, spent a day in Portsmouth, walked to Pembridge Church and back, to Priory Farm and back, and to the shops where they spent their pocket money. Florence was forced to take her shoes to a cobbler in Ryde, which was a five-mile trek but she did not feel tired afterwards. She was also obliged to mend the holes in her clothes herself because she did not go home early, as Parthe had. The girls drew and read Shakespeare, and any criticism of the holiday was directed at cousin Alfie, who had been so idle that they had to cancel three outings as a punishment; also that she had a painful boil on her arm and with the poultice on she could not write nicely, and that people smoked too much there. It was a balanced healthy holiday of fresh air, exercise, sea bathing, and intellectual pursuits.

Sea bathing became popular in England in the mid-eighteenth century, notably at Scarborough and Brighton. The prescribed method of bathing was in the morning, on an empty stomach, and after the bowels had emptied. It was recommended for stimulating and reviving the constitution, as being beneficial in glandular and lymphatic complaints such as scrofula; for alleviating gout, rheumatism, some skin diseases, and melancholy. Sea bathers were expected to emerge feeling a healthy glow, then either rub themselves down with a flesh brush or take some lively exercise. If they emerged feeling headachy and lethargic, sea-bathing was doing them more harm than good and they should immediately stop it.

In October 1834 Florence, Parthe and Betsy [possibly one of the Nightingales' servants] were again in the Isle of Wight, this time at Cowes. Shortly afterwards they were joined by Aunt Mai's three younger children, Blanche 6, Shore 3, and baby Bertha, their nurse Miss White, and servant Mary. Flo and Bertha shared a room overlooking the sea. The sea shore and the hillside were dotted with charming houses and West Cowes at that time was described as 'a delightful summer residence down by the sea-side or westward of the castle, or up the hill peering over the shore'. The sea was easily accessible from bathing machines parked near the castle, and there were also some much sought after hot salt water baths. The real charm of Cowes was the never-ending bustle of expensive private English and foreign yachts, and steamers bringing in the day-trippers.

There was no danger of anyone overheating. The house was bitterly cold and at times Florence's hands were so numb she could barely hold a pen. Nevertheless they followed a daily routine, getting up just after 7 o'clock and preparing cold salt water. Every morning and evening Florence had her ankles and feet bathed and rubbed in it. At great expense - sixpence a week - she hired a tub so that she could stand in it and pour a bucket of the water over herself. That took just over an hour, during which Miss White and Shore also had salt water thrown over them. This was known as the Pail Bath.

Fanny had instructed Miss White to take baths three times a week, and Florence twice a week at 88°F. Florence grumbled that this was much too cold considering both the weather and that her mother had earlier told her they should be at 95 or 96°F. Betsy was also bathing three times a week at 95°F and was taking sea water internally which, Florence noted with relief, didn't make her sick. These baths were probably taken at Jacob Hewitt's three-storey bath house, which he had established in 1790 and offered, 'Hot plunging and salt water baths'. Hewitt's also kept a sedan chair for the use of its customers and a list of lodging houses.

Florence wrote home frequently, keeping her mother up to date with all the news and in return receiving news, chickens and seed cakes, for which she was very grateful because everything in Cowes was so expensive. At the end of the holiday Blanche and Betsy, who had both been unwell, were much restored.

Chapter II
A Highly Popular Amusement: Malvern, 1848

In September 1846 Florence reported to her adored cousin, William Shore Smith, that, 'Mrs Fowler has been at Malvern a great establishment for the Water Cure, trying it on upon herself, though she is quite well. Example is better than, etc. The doctor is a bearer of the word only & not &c.' Anne Fowler, who had an enquiring and useful mind, and her husband, Dr Richard Fowler, an elderly physician at the Salisbury Infirmary, were family friends. Flo jovially endorsed Mrs Fowler's trip to Malvern, the references to the proverb 'Example is better than precept' and 'the doctor being the bearer of the word only', reinforcing her opinion that doctors would teach people more effectively by example rather than by merely telling them what to do.

By 1846 Malvern had been a tranquil, healthy tourist resort for over a hundred years but it was only in 1842, with the arrival of hydropathic doctors James Wilson and James Gully, that the Water Cure was introduced on the sound principles of its founder, Vincenz Priessnitz. The two Malvern doctors quickly achieved status, fame and wealth, and attracted many aristocratic and well-known personalities to their establishments. The visitors, who were listed in the Worcester newspapers, read like a combination of *Burke's Peerage* and *Who's Who*. For example, *The Worcester Herald* of 14th October 1848 announced that Mrs and Miss Nightingale were in Malvern.

Florence described to Parthe how they took the train from Birmingham to Spetchley, on the outskirts of Worcester, then travelled the twelve miles by road to Malvern. As they approached the village, 'we drove through a Triumphal Arch of wet sheets & an avenue of flannels to the Foley Arms - & went to bed, I between curtains &

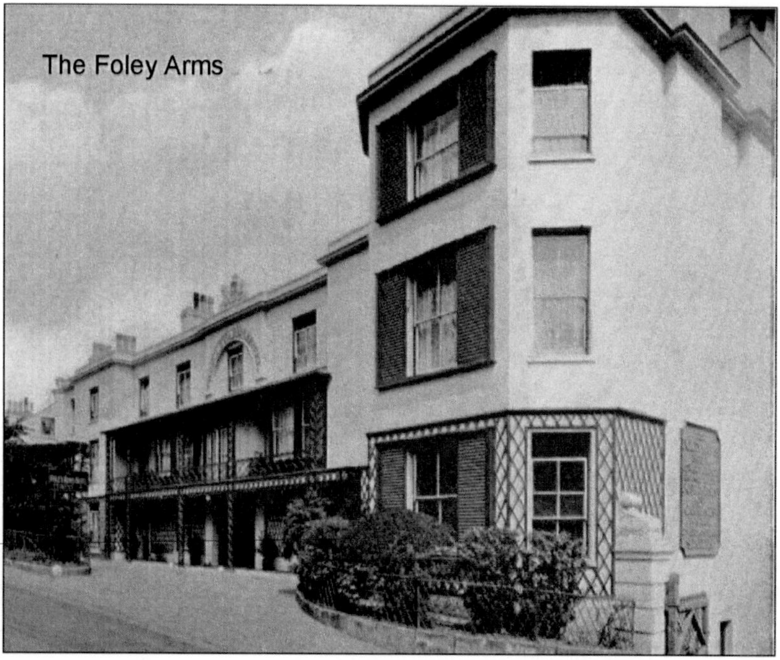

Mama upon sofas directly. This morn we sent for Gully & Mama was so taken in by him that I was obliged to tell him I had a father living.

She is positively beginning his treatment but he says that even I must be as gradual as possible. I liked him too very much, tho' he didn't agree with me (a great merit in me) but Mama thought his head like Napoleon's, because he did think like her, I mean. However that may be, she has been and bought his book directly. He considers us as very mild females and to be treated very mild I liked him too very much....' Dr Gully recommended his book *The Water Cure in Chronic Disease* to his patients because from it they might learn the causes of their ailment, the treatment, and the likely outcome. The book ended up in Florence's book case.

With her prescription from Dr Gully, the next day Florence began her treatment. She told Parthe the full horrors of the Water Cure. 'This morning the operation began; a young woman roused me out of bed, set me down, with only a small girdle about my loins, like John the

Baptist, before a great tub, & seizing a dripping towel out of it, began a violent assault on my back, while, in order I believe to divert my attention, she gave me another heap of dripping linen, counselling me to do the same to my chest, which of course, I carefully avoided doing. She then popped my feet into cold water, & proceeded with the same operation on my legs and said she'd come again at 12 o'clock. Mama is to have a very mild infusion of the same process. Then I ran up to the top of the hill before breakfast. The weather here is like summer; we are going out on another campaign after lodgings... a hard job for the place is full and we are difficult...'

The search for lodgings in crowded Malvern was eventually successful and mother and daughter moved in to South Villa, next to Holyrood House, Dr Gully's hydropathic establishment for men, and a short walk above the 'wicked old church' - 'wicked' because it did not have a daily service. The view from South Villa is a spectacular panorama across to Birmingham and Worcester to the north, the Cotswolds, Bredon Hill, and the Severn Plain to the east, and Upton and Tewkesbury to the south. Almost as soon as they had moved in snow fell and the weather turned coldly wintry for over a week. Florence thought that Malvern could be quite lovely with a bit of

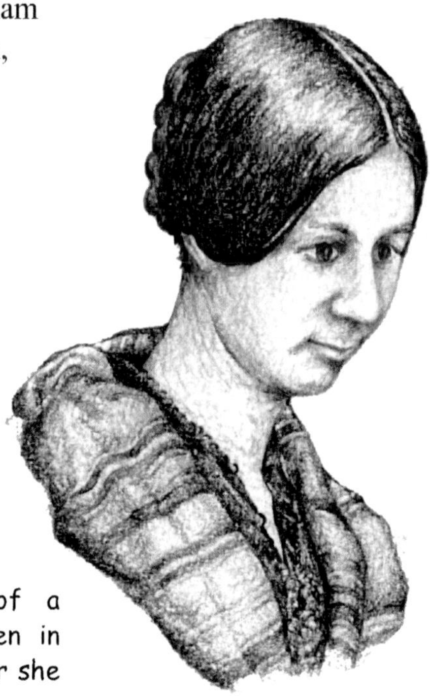

A copy by Peter Lloyd of a photograph of Florence taken in Berlin on 1849, the year after she came to Malvern.

Map of Great Malvern

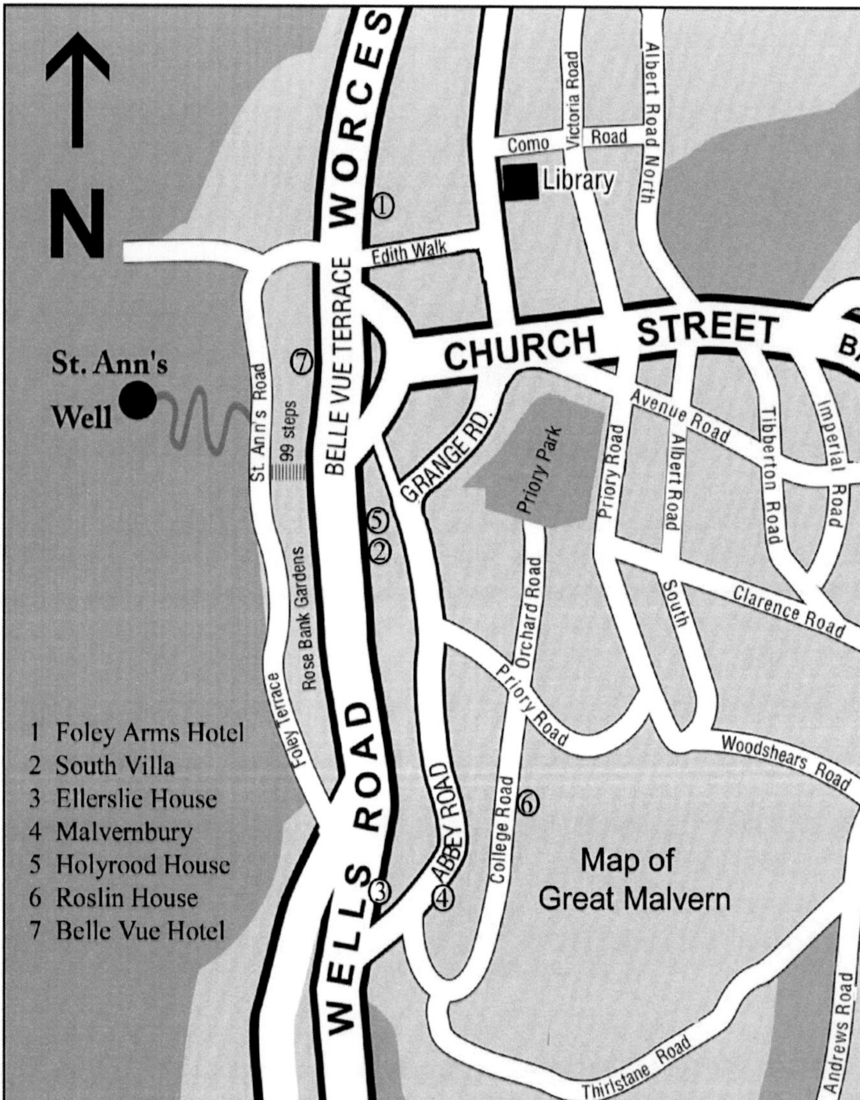

fine weather and when it came she was enchanted with the vibrant little village, which she later described as her 'first love'. She described the hills as being like the Pyrenees and wrote to her father of her early-morning rising and solo escapade up the hills. 'I & the little birds saw the sun rise from the heights this morning & not even

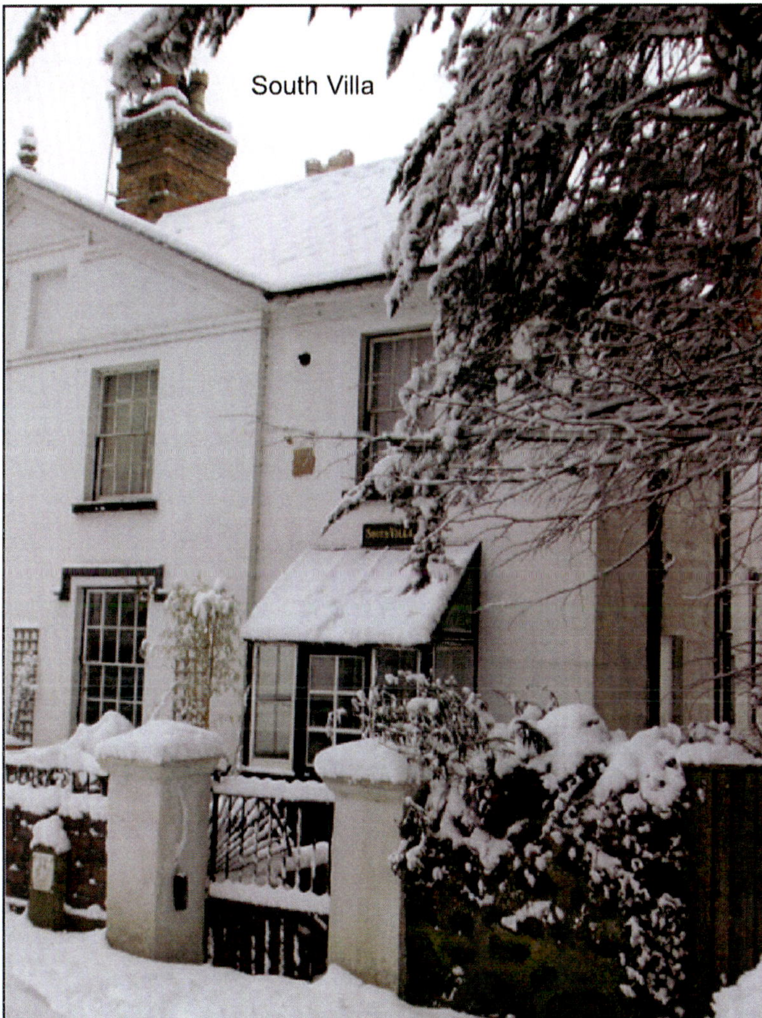

Malvern was full and it was difficult to find lodgings, so Fanny and Florence were pleased to find South Villa in Wells Road, near the centre of the village. It snowed.

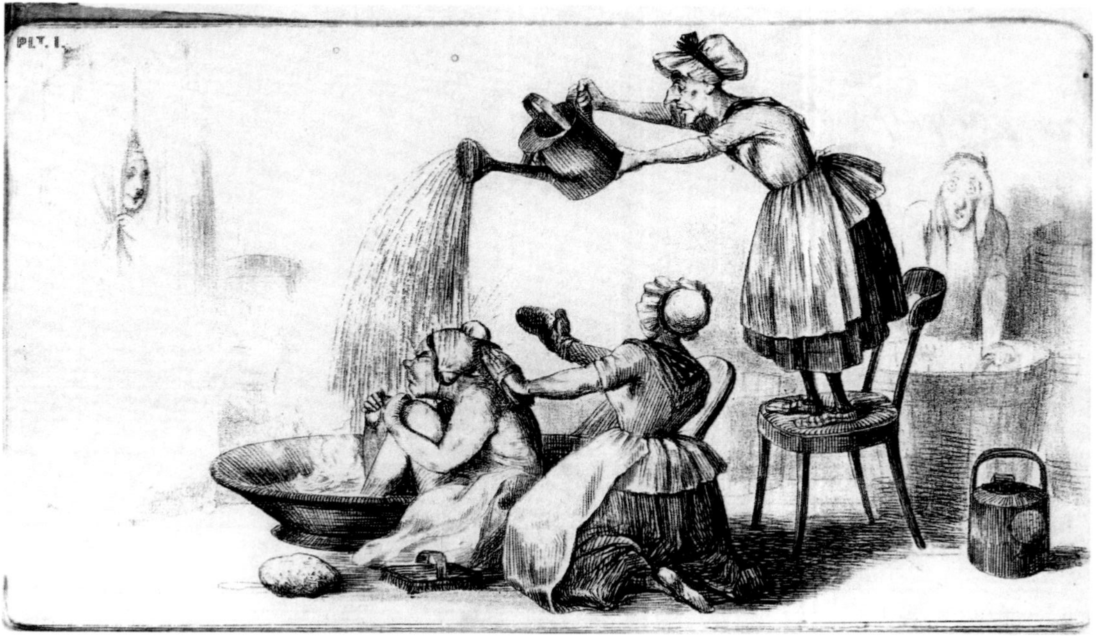

'This is a prelude to the full Bath, a considerate mitigation for delicate constitutions. The Patient is watered till she feels strangled, or Hydrophobially affected, and then rubbed till the Body is sore...Horse hair Gloves, we strongly recommend... which will be found highly beneficial to all ladies troubled with old Maidish peculiarities. It might cure if any one could be found to use it often enough.'

'from *The Sure Water Cure*, Messrs Fores, 44 Piccadilly, London (July 1843)

Picture and text courtesy of Roger Hall-Jones.

Early risers climbed the hills before the donkeys were awake.

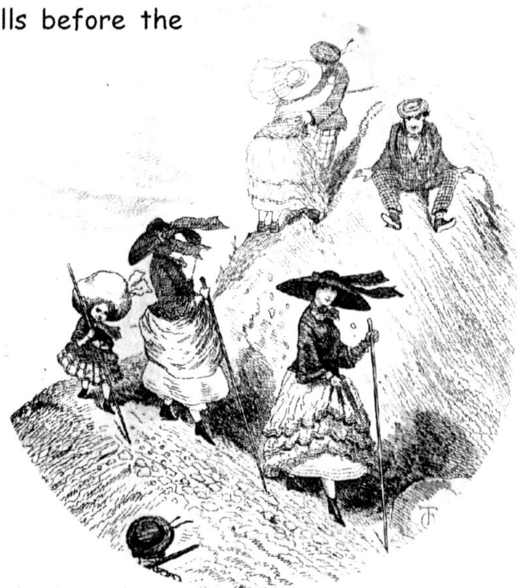

the donkeys were awake – excepting me. The Severn was enormously swollen so that the vast plain looked all cut up with rivers, but I suppose I saw the Avon as well & Worcester Cathedral seemed to stand a little island in the midst of overflowing waters.'

The regime of early to bed, early rising, and exercise strengthened Florence's constitution to the point where, after two weeks, she could endure the brandy and soda of the water cure, the Douche. Florence captured the moment of the Douche in a letter to Parthe. 'My treatment is as follows, if you want to know: packing in the morning; dripping sheet after douche at noon, a new & horrible instrument of torture. You go down to the douche house, where you hear a series of little yells & squeals proceeding from the victims along the line & sometimes a prolonged howl. You go into your own den & descend into a deep well. Above are three pipes of 2", 3", 4" bore, about ten feet above your head. And there you stand, stark staring naked (& mad too) like Eve in the Garden of Eden receiving some punishment from the Angels – it is so like a natural castigation – the woman continually peeping thro' a window at the top, like Nebuchadnezzar to see that Daniel does not escape from the lions – which takes you just in the small of your back... and the woman says, if you ask her why people don't escape - 'Ah miss, we has 'em there. If it weren't for the shock, they'd be twice as cold; they're obliged to stand under to warm theirselves.'

They had a footbath in the afternoons, and nightly fomentations.

Their dear friends Charles and Selena Bracebridge were also in Malvern, both very much under the weather. Selena looked ill but said she was better and Florence was so frightened about Charles that she had a word with Dr Gully about his condition. Gully shook his head and made a comment to Florence which he hoped she would not repeat. Two years later, in 1850, Charles Bracebridge was at the Prussian spa of Pyrmont, searching for a cure, and he went there the following year as well. The Bracebridges must have recovered their health because they accompanied Florence to Scutari and the Crimea 1854-55.

In spas where the drinking of mineralised water was the main treatment, the treatment usually took place early in the morning on an empty stomach. That left the rest of the day for finding interesting things to do. Malvern was essentially a bathing and wrapping spa, the treatments lasting throughout the day so leaving little time for entertainment and excursions. Thus in Malvern in 1848 there was little to do in the way of entertainment apart from walking, talking, donkey riding, the occasional ball, or listening to the Rhine String Band at St Ann's Well or along Belle Vue Terrace.

Unless they wished to remain incognito, arrivals at spas wrote their name and their lodging address in the Visitors Book which, at Malvern, was kept at the Royal Library. Any friends also visiting the spa could thus find you, and you them. The Nightingales did not wish to be found at Malvern, so they were quite dismayed when, within two weeks of their arrival, the Dean of St Asaph and his friends, Mr and Mrs Scudamore, turned up on the doorstep. Florence wrote despairingly to her father '...heaven knows how they found us out - & asking us to dine & sleep – but we said we were too ill.' Later, however, when the improving treatment put them in a better frame of mind for meeting people, Florence wrote to Parthe about some of the people they met. She had become acquainted with, 'a poor little Estonian exile here of three & twenty, from the island of Oesel (where's that, stoopid?) who is living, or rather dying, here by giving lessons... ', and had discovered that the Ladies Proby were in Malvern. They were, 'old relations of Mrs J. Mackenzies, recommended to us & we are positively going to put on our best caps to tea with them tonight. Gully drank tea with us last night. He is always interesting ...' and added that he 'wd make an admirable adviser but a bad friend – however this is very ungrateful, as he has been very kind to me.'

Florence and Fanny's arrival was sandwiched between the arrival of the future poet laureate Alfred Tennyson's the previous month, and the departure of Tennyson's elderly poet laureate predecessor, William Wordsworth, for London the following month. Florence chanced upon Tennyson one day, and related to her dear friend and former suitor Richard Monckton Milnes how, 'Your friend, Alfred Tennyson was there with a skin so tender he walked backwards whenever the wind was north or east and that was generally. He was sadly contumacious, smoking vile tobacco in a long pipe till Dr Gully told him that it coarsened his imagination and made him write bad poetry.'

Apart from brisk walking or hill climbing, outdoor exercise was limited as the weather turned to snow. 'Cold weather?' she wrote to Parthe, after five weeks at Malvern. 'My dear friend! Drive us away? To people who have lived under a Douche which rains small hail stones, cold weather's a fool, frost's my natural fur, and snow I thatch my head with. Ice I keep in my waistcoat pocket... We've a deep snow on the ground, what do you think of that? I have not seen a snow these two years and stood at the window like a child this morning to see the red fuchsias nodding at each other under the heavy white covering...'

At the end of November, after seven weeks in Malvern she wrote home, 'I get up much earlier now & am out before it's light at 7 o'clock. I like to see the fires lighting up in the houses & think how uncomfortable I am (outside). A man who is uncomfortable may be, if he chooses, in a much higher state of existence than a comfortable man.' And then Mrs and Miss Nightingale returned to their winter home at Embley. Almost immediately Florence summed up her experience. '..... we are both much the better for our ablutions. I have done penance twice a day in wet sheets and my companion, notwithstanding the villainous weather, has fought bravely through the whole series of torments – doughy packings and many minor tortures – and there is no question as to our crowns of martyrdom. I would gladly have put off the operation till milder weather, but Dr. Gully would not hear of it, preferring the winter for his afflictions. So, if you have still any intention of submitting yourself to him, now's your time. It is hard work, requiring all your time, much faith and an enthusiastic spirit. We have many friends in the neighbourhood whose blandishments we were obliged to resist, but, fortunately here at Malvern to interfere with our operations, society and water cure being quite incompatible.'

She had been prescribed the Packing in the morning, the Douche followed by the Dripping Sheet at midday, Foot baths in the afternoon, and nightly fomentations. No wonder she complained that the worst of the water cure was that it took up all of one's time, and it may have been as a result of this visit that she memorably described the water cure as 'a highly popular amusement within the last few years amongst athletic invalids who have felt the tedium vitae, and those indefinite diseases which a large income and unbounded leisure are so well calculated to produce.'

Chapter III
Sedation and Stimulation: How the Water Cure Works

The application of water to the body can do two things: sedate the stressed and stimulate the stagnant. Many wealthy Victorians were so over-indulgent with food and alcohol, and under-indulgent in exercise, that their circulation was poor; they suffered chronically from [among other things] constipation, indigestion, obesity and lethargy. Their blood was like a sea in the stomach, which stoically macerated the endless meals sent its way. The blood was given no chance to escape to the head and limbs to keep the whole body working and in good health. The blood needed to circulate. When you get into a hot bath the skin, of its own accord, turns pink. This is because the blood automatically moves slowly to the skin to try to cool the body. When you get into cold water, such as the sea, the blood automatically moves gently inwards, to try to keep the vital organs warm. Knowing this basic principle of how the body responds to temperature, slothful circulation could easily be improved.

The Packing

The Packing lowers the circulation, reduces excess blood in some organs and distributes it to organs that have a deficiency. It was the first treatment of a spa patient's day, and admirably described by Richard Lane. '...at six the bath attendant appeared with what seemed like a coil of linen cable, and a gigantic can of water, and it was some comfort to pretend not to be in the least degree apprehensive. I was ordered out of bed and all the clothes taken off. Two blankets were then spread upon the mattress, and half over the pillow, and the wet sheet unfolded and placed upon them. Having stretched my length upon it and lying on my back, the man quickly and most adroitly folded it – first on one side and then on the other, and closely round the neck, and the same with the two blankets, by which time I was warm, and sufficiently composed to ask how the sheet was prepared of the proper degree of dampness. (I was told that being soaked well, it is held by two persons – one at each end, and pulled and twisted until water has ceased to drop). Two more doubled blankets were then put upon me, and each in turn tucked most carefully round the neck, and under me. Upon this the down bed was placed, and over all another sheet or counterpane was secured at all sides and under the chin, to complete this hermetical sealing. By this time I was sure of being fast asleep in five minutes.' One man, who had not experienced this process first hand, shuddered with disgust as he explained the process to Lane; but Lane found the 'mild atmosphere of warm vapour' so comfortable and relaxing that he looked forward to it every morning.

When cold water is applied to the body, the skin automatically creates a warm layer between the skin and the water. This is why immersion in cold water, such as the sea, feels less cold after a few seconds. We say it's because we're 'getting used to the water'. With

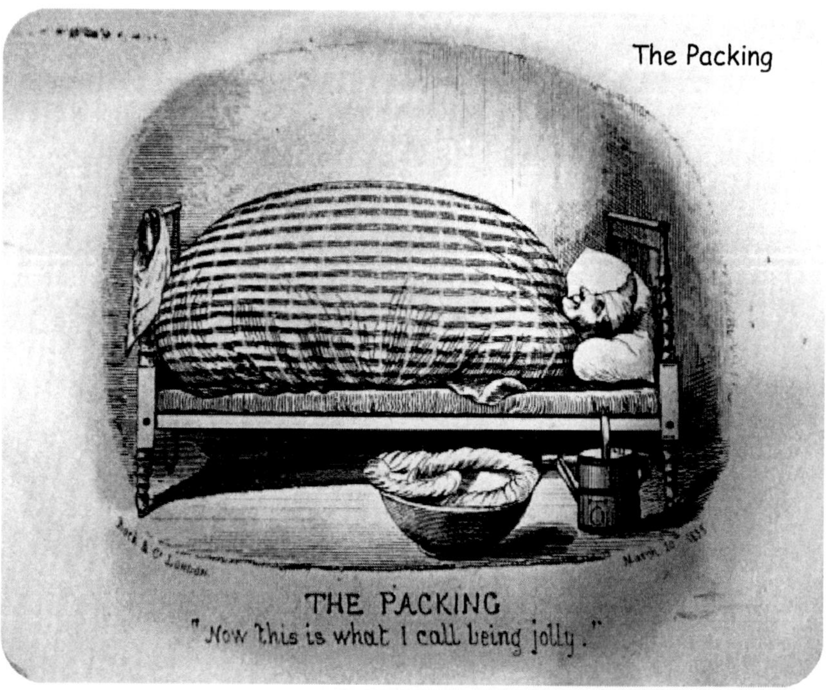

The Packing

the Packing, the initial coldness of the sheet sends the blood inwards; the warm layer created between the skin and the sheet then brings the blood back to the surface. Packing for more than half an hour has a soporific sedative effect, so a patient who was only to be stimulated was removed from the sheets after 10 or 15 minutes. For best advantage from this treatment the Packing was followed immediately by the cold dripping sheet, to stimulate the stagnant.

The Douche

In his *Life at the Water Cure*, Richard Lane, who was a patient of Dr Wilson's, described taking the Douche for the first time. 'It was an anxious point with me to take it discreetly, - according to the Doctor's directions. First on the back between the shoulders, then down the spine, then on the right shoulder, and on the whole of the right side; never on the head, until, having received it one full minute, I placed my hands (the fingers interlaced) over my head, and so broke the compact column into a delicious shower of foam. The fall of water is nearly twenty feet from the cistern. A pipe descends about two feet from the cistern, tapering downwards to concentrate the force of the fall. With me the re-action was immediate. On going to the dressing room I was instantly hot. The attendant said that I shone "like a new guinea". Had I a headache? - No. Was I giddy? - No. Warm? - Am I not? All was perfection!' He added that a broken chair in the corner of the dressing room was the result of a stout lady clambering on to it to reduce the height of the column of water. Weight and water had caused a collapse and a great fall, from which it took the lady a week to recover. Was the water cold? Lane heard a story of a man being wounded on the shoulder by a falling icicle but the water was so cold that he didn't feel a thing.

The Dripping Sheet

This is used to prepare skin that is unaccustomed to being in contact with water below body temperature. The shock of the cold water is counteracted by friction rubbing of the skin. The result is that the blood-vessels of the skin contract in the first instance, and then relax,

The Douche was the brandy and soda of the Water Cure

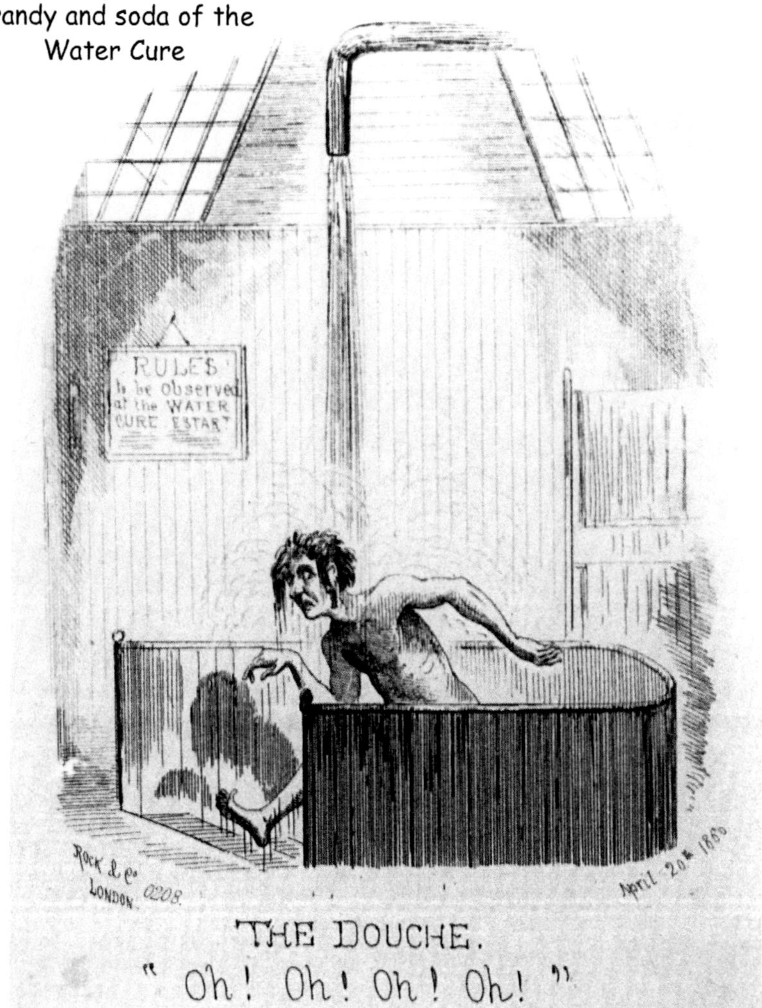

allowing more blood into the blood vessels. The friction rub, followed by exercise, ensures that the blood stays in the skin, creating a healthy glow rather than a pasty pastel. It also stimulates the body's circulatory and nervous systems, and reduces irritation in the internal organs. '...it takes off languor, gives alacrity to mind and limb, clears away intellectual and moral cloudiness, at the same time that it generates appetite, removes thirst, causes expulsion of flatulence &c.'

John Smedley described how he spread a mackintosh on the bedroom floor before beginning the process. 'A cold dripping sheet at any time of the day when fatigued is very refreshing.... it is easily managed by putting the wet sheet like a cloak, and with the hands out rubbing and drawing the sheet backwards and forwards over the back. I cannot speak too highly of the effects of the dripping sheet'. By the 1870s the 'Malvern bathing-sheet' was recommended when a dripping sheet was required. It consisted of 2½ yards of a coarse kind of canvas two yards wide that was hauled from a bucket of water, and thrown over the patient, who was rubbed very briskly before being rubbed down with a dry Malvern sheet.

The Foot Bath

The palms and soles have more nerves and blood vessels than any other part of the body of the same size, which is why they are so ticklish. Hand and foot baths can relieve pain, weary weakness, and fidgets. Foot baths also act on the digestive organs, relieving nausea, sinking and gnawing feelings, and flatulence. [Today, reflexologists and masseurs know the extent of the relation between foot and stomach.] The shock of the water and the friction draws blood to the feet and warms them up. '...a cold foot bath of twelve or fifteen minutes, followed by a walk of half an hour, is the most certain way to warm the feet that can be devised,' advised Dr Gully. If a patient was unable to walk, or found walking difficult, mustard was added to the cold water and a dry friction rub with brushes or rough towels followed the soak. Charles Darwin had this treatment when he first came to Malvern in 1849 to take the water cure under Dr Gully. 'At 12 o'clock I put my feet for 10 minutes in cold water with a little mustard & they are violently rubbed by my man...' John Smedley's recipe was to walk about in five or six inches of cold water or stand in a tub stamping the feet, for five or six minutes, rub them dry and take some exercise. He said he walked in snow or on wet grass for up to half an hour, or removed his shoes and socks and walked in the brook – replacing the garments without drying his feet. Smedley recommended Foot Baths as a tonic because they reduce headache, draw blood to the feet, and can be used by anyone – even those in perfect health.

Fomentations

This was similar to the Packing. A mackintosh was spread over the bed and two blankets spread on top. Then the patient, either completely undressed or only the trunk undressed, lay on the blanket. A fomenting flannel, i.e a flannel wrung out with hot water, was placed under the back and another over the chest and bowels. One side of the blanket was drawn over the patient, the arms put down, a hot can laid on, the other side of the blanket drawn over, then the mackintosh. The patient lay quietly for three quarters of an hour to an hour. This treatment was a mild sedative and relaxant and useful in afflictions of the stomach, chest and liver and in pains, cramps and headaches.

The water cure can cure, but if a patient returns home and resumes a stressful and unhealthy lifestyle, the symptoms will recur, as the friends of recidivist Alfred Tennyson found. 'Alfred is also here, having just emerged from the water-process at Malvern. He now drinks a bottle of wine a day, and smokes as before; a sure way to throw back in a week or two all the benefit (if benefit there were) which resulted from many weeks of privation and penance.'

Chapter IV
The Hospitals of Europe: Carlsbad, Franzensbad and Harrogate

One August, c.1838, Fanny Nightingale took Parthe and Florence to Carlsbad, the hospital of Europe in the early nineteenth century and famous for its Sprudel, a spout of hot water of 73°C, which was saline and rich in iron and carbon dioxide. This was a town for the ill, not for the well, so all visitors were under the instruction of a medical adviser. It could be fatal for an invalid to take advice from another spa patient, because the water at one spa may not be the right water for a patient suffering from a different, or even the same, disease. There were many cases of people dying through the imprudent use of mineral waters. Fanny had consulted Dr Weber in London who had recommended Carlsbad followed by Franzensbad, a combination widely recommended by English and German doctors. Carlsbad waters were recommended for digestive problems, gravel and stones, blood disorders, constipation, ailments of the mesentery, liver and spleen, and was particularly good for women's problems.

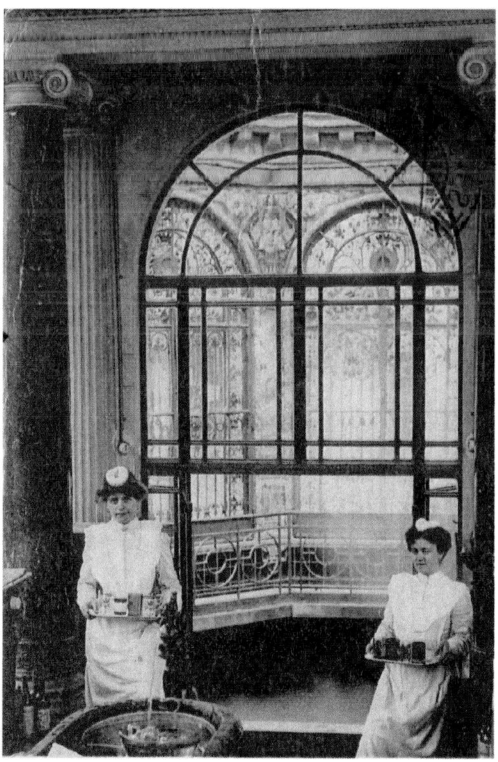

At German spas, pristine dippers served mineral water to the invalids.

Drinking was done early on an empty stomach, so most people were at the fountain by 6am. Dippers filled the glasses and the water was sipped slowly, with gentle exercise of 15 minutes between each glass. Generally, invalids drank five or six 6oz beakers of the recommended water over the course of one and a half to two hours. If patients became constipated they took Carlsbad salts or a saline water. The toilets were nearby. Breakfast was about an hour after the last glass of water.

Parthe, who loved mixing with the crowds of water bibbers, chose to drink every morning at the Theresienbrunn, named in 1798 in honour of the Empress Maria Theresa, and which was in a rotunda at the foot of a hill. Ladies preferred this spring because it was set in a garden and because it was dedicated to a lady. Between glasses or while they were waiting for the waters to 'work', drinkers usually paced monotonously up and down under a covered wooden building. But here the ladies could take the zig-zag paths to the top of the hill, which was covered with flowers and plants. At the top was the König von England [King of England] Hotel, which had commanding views over the whole valley. Alternatively the ladies gossiped among themselves or, if they preferred quiet, took themselves off to the elegant Salle de Sprudel with its flower parterre and comfortable Ottomans. This room was 100 feet long, with eleven large windows, mirrors and arabesque paintings on the walls, and a polished wood floor. Florence could not face the early morning crowds and music, so did not go to the Theresienbrunn.

On 27th August they finished their treatment at Carlsbad. Florence had gone there unable to sleep well and with indigestion and weakness, but she felt much better after treatment and Dr Meissner confirmed that she was indeed better. Fanny had a Crisis* of sickness but felt better afterwards and the pains in her legs had disappeared.

*The Crisis was a physical sign that the invalid was on the mend, and might be characterised by a boil, a rash, headache, sickness or diarrhoea, or generally feeling out of sorts.

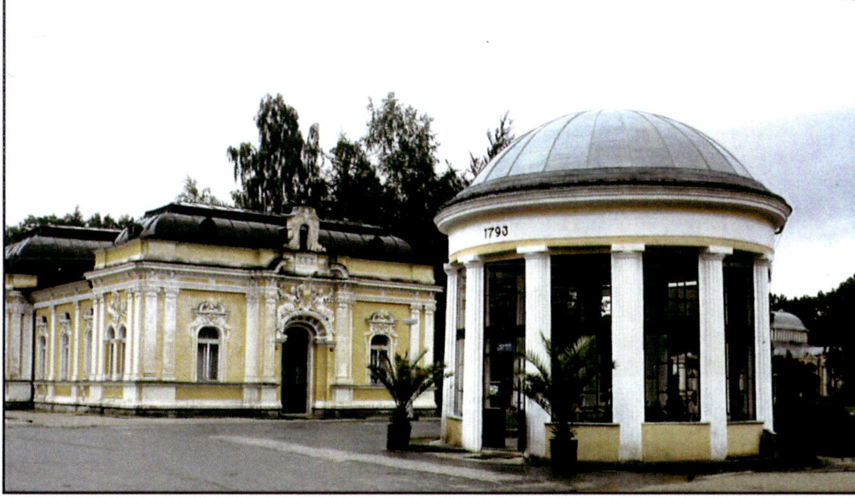

The Franzens-quelle, Franzensbad

Only Parthe needed to go to Franzensbad. For two weeks she was to take baths as a tonic, or three weeks if they seemed to be doing her good. Dr Granville described the town as monotonous and dreary 'where nature seems sanative without being smiling', adding that it stood a poor chance of success when its rival spas were so picturesque, inspiring and enchanting. Florence thought the town hideous. The chief spring there was the Franzens-quelle [Francis Spring], containing iron, Glauber salt and carbonic acid [carbon dioxide] and was used in cases of debility. Parthe's baths would have been taken about two hours after breakfast, with a temperature ranging between 90 and 98°F. There was a choice of chalybeate water baths, mud baths or gas baths for a variety of ailments, so we cannot ascertain what Parthe's problems were.

Parthe did not regain her health and throughout the summer of 1839 she became increasingly weak and thin. In May Florence wrote to a friend that Parthe was not very strong so was staying away from London, and in September she remarked how she wished the family had spent another winter in Italy because Parthe had been so well there. The Nightingales were living rough at Embley, where building and decorating work was in progress, so Parthe was packed off to Harrogate by her parents in September, accompanied by Aunt Mai and the Parker family.* She would be warm there and could take the mineral waters. Because of its wet days and cold nights the season did not really begin at Harrogate until the first half of August, by which time the poorer classes had departed and the seasonal higher prices were introduced. Harrogate's strong chalybeate [iron-bearing] spring was discovered in the late sixteenth century and Harrogate was the first place in England to be designated a spa, after its namesake Spa in Belgium. Chalybeate water, discernible by its orange sediment and taste of rusty nails, was used frequently by anaemic women and those unable to conceive. The iron was easily assimilable by the body and, if it caused constipation, was used in conjunction with saline water. Dr Adam Hunter always prescribed Harrogate's saline-chalybeate water, 'In all female weaknesses.'

Harrogate was famous not only for its chalybeate water but also for its saline and stinking sulphur waters which, between them, treated glandular diseases, scrofulous ailments, biliary derangements, constipation, skin diseases such as boils, liver complaints and rheumatic disorders. The recommended daily dose of sulphur water at that time was two glasses of three quarters of a pint each [12 fluid ounces], with a 20 minute interval between the glasses, each day for three to six weeks. In Germany the glasses were much smaller, at only 4 fluid ounces, which was considered far better for patients. Drinking was done early so between half past six and eight o'clock patients could be seen swarming from their lodgings towards their prescribed spout.

After her treatment here Parthenope remained weak, but water treatment can have a delayed reaction, as Florence found after her 1848 visit to Malvern, and by January 1840 Parthe was much stronger. She was almost certainly anaemic: an intolerance of cold weather, tiredness and lethargy are all symptoms of anaemia, which is usually the result of iron deficiency that in women was often the result

* Mr Parker was one of the Lords of the Treasury

of heavy periods. A letter from Parthe to her mother c.1858 and shortly after her marriage talks of having an early period which 'does not signify small events' perhaps a reference to a miscarriage or not being pregnant.

In the autumn of 1848 Parthe was advised to go again to Carlsbad to take the Water Cure but because of riots breaking out there she stayed at home. Three years later, in August 1851, and accompanied by Fanny, Parthe was again taking the waters at the German spas, apparently for three months for gynaecological problems. Flo wrote to her at Franzensbad commiserating that she hated the town quite so much. She wrote later to say how sorry she was that Parthe was not making more progress with the treatment. In December 1858, six months after her marriage, Parthe had a miscarriage. She never had children, so perhaps her medical problems were mainly blood-related and gynaecological.

On 3rd May 1852 Florence accompanied her 54-year-old Aunt Mai to Harrogate, where she was to take the waters. Florence wrote immediately to her mother telling how, when they arrived, they took lodgings opposite the church, as usual, on the understanding that the house would not be painted while they were staying there. It was the start of the season and there seemed to be a lot of painting going on at the time. But no sooner had they moved in than painting began. Although they could not smell paint, they thought they ought to be able to and, worried what Mrs Nightingale and the world would say if they knew that they were staying in a house that was being painted, '... we packed up our things in a rage and trundled out' and found alternative lodgings at a guinea a week. But then they worried what Mrs Nightingale would think of them lodging at a guinea a week, and as painting had also begun in that house, 'We bundled out again and, after hunting all Harrogate through, high, low and middle, we have settled ourselves at a very superior lodging, Mrs. Wright's, York Place... But alas! It is £2 /5 a week – very different from our last. And it is in Middle Harrogate, and we can't hear the ecclesiastical clock strike. We have got a window and two daughters plus a widow.' 'We are quite satisfied with our lodgings & drink the water with enthusiasm,' Flo wrote.

After the early morning drinking the rest of the day was free and Florence was hoping to take Aunt Mai to Castle Howard 'for a lark', but it was raining,'... & not before it was wanted – for the dust covered the table in the old bow, as you sat with closed windows. I never saw anything like it except in Egypt. The country round here is all sandstone, so that the dust is not a fine impalpable powder, but like large brickbats flying about. I dare say we shall have a month's rain more.' However they did get the water drinking over early one morning and spent the day in York. On 13th May Florence wrote thanking her mother for sending her enough money to cover her expenses, '...having paid all our bills handsome, & made beasts of ourselves at all the houses of entertainment.' Florence's expenses for eight days were £1 8s 8 d for the lodgings and 11s 8d for board, slightly less than two guineas for the week.

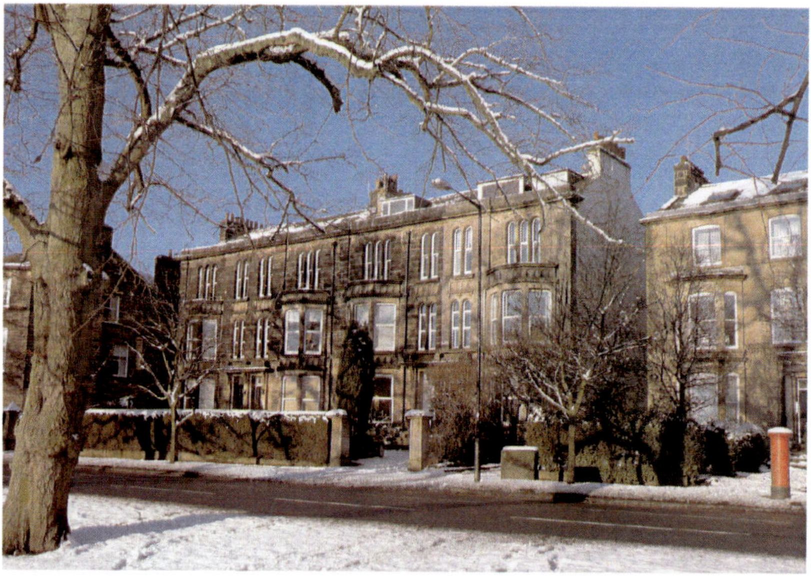

Florence and Aunt Mai stayed at Mrs Wright's very superior lodging here at York Place

Chapter V
Umberslade Bethesda

In July 1850 Florence was staying with the Bracebridges at Pyrmont; from there she would head for Düsseldorf. W.E.N had an eye problem, so she suggested that he write all the details of the problem and send them to her at Düsseldorf. She would then take the details to the famous oculist Friederich Hermann de Leuw, who practised at Gräfrath, a village two hours away from Düsseldorf, and get his opinion on the problem. Florence suspected that her father suffered the same problem as his sister, Aunt Mai, who had already forwarded her details. Florence managed to see Dr de Leuw in August; he thought the eye inflammation was external, rather than the more severe internal, but could not be sure without a consultation. However the eye problem was soon supported sympathetically by a severe bout of constipation and W.E.N consulted Dr Gully, who proposed a week at Malvern. After her lengthy stay at Malvern three years earlier Florence was not sure that one week was enough. She wrote to her father. 'Dear Papa, I doubt whether it is possible for even a water cure to produce any difference whatever at the end of one week. Is Gully satisfied that you should try only a week & then come away? I stayed seven weeks & found little difference till after I came away. If it is the noise which you dislike, I think it would do me a great deal of good to have a little water cure after my measles, & I should like to come & take a little lodging with you very much, dear Papa...'

Dr Gully would have made a visit to Malvern undeniably attractive, but there were two reasons why Malvern was unsuitable. Firstly, if they went to Gully's they would have had to stay in separate lodgings because at that time Dr Gully was only operating one establishment, Holyrood House, which was solely for male patients. Secondly, Malvern was a noisy building site. Since the mid-1840s, when land to the north, south and east of the village had become available for building, new, sweeping roads lined with large, handsome houses had been built for new, wealthy residents, hordes of seasonal visitors, and the trade and servant classes who were needed to serve them. Also, messy and noisy excavations may already have been under way for Dr Gully's new hydropathic establishment next door to Holyrood House.*

On a snowy Monday, 5th January1852, Florence accompanied her father to Umberslade Hall in the village of Tanworth-in-Arden, Warwickshire, where they both intended to regain their health. They arrived at 6.30 in the evening and immediately Florence went to see the doctor, Edward Johnson, to explain her father's ailments. At 7 o'clock they sat down to tea with the other residents. These included the Johnson family, consisting of Dr Edward Johnson, his wife Fanny,

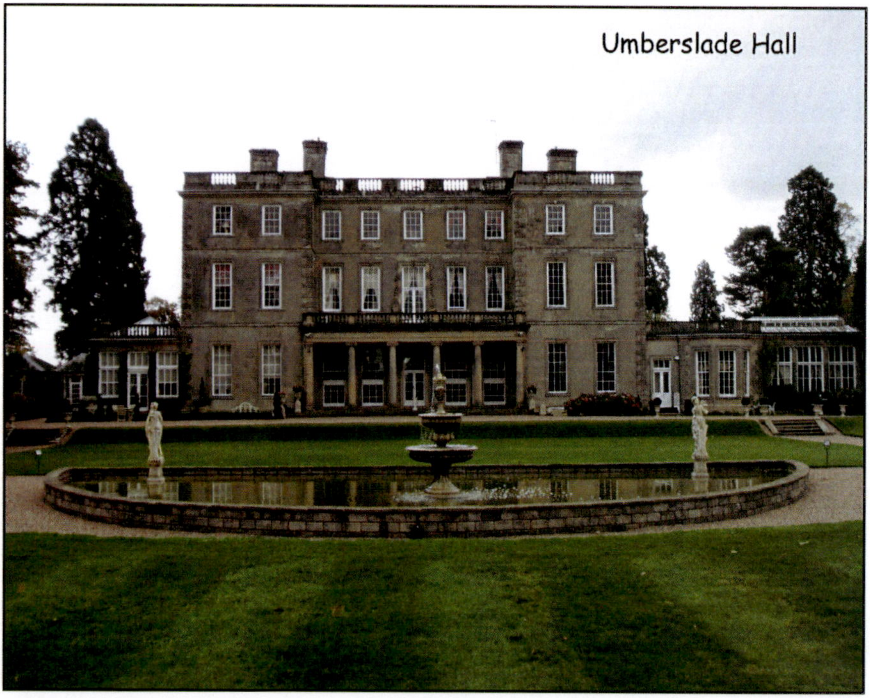
Umberslade Hall

* The village was growing so quickly that an Act of Parliament was passed in September 1851 granting town status.

their four sons and two nieces, and five other water cure patients: Mr and Mrs Ford, two gentlemen, and an unmarried lady. None was from polished society, as Florence pointed out. Mrs Ford, she observed, sat with her hands between her knees and 'Mrs Johnson does not h'aspirate her haitches.' Florence wrote to her cousin Hilary, '.... Poor Cassandra* has found an unexpected ally in a young surgeon of a London hospital, a son of Dr Johnson who sits next to Papa at the table d'hôte. The account he gives of the nurses beats everything that even I know of. This young prophet says they are all drunkards without exception, Sisters and all, and that there are but two nurses whom the surgeon can trust to give the patients their medicines. I thought you would be pleased to hear how bad they are, so I tell you.'**

After tea they had a consultation with the doctor. He was sure he could restore W.E.N's health to what it had been six months earlier but insulted Florence by describing her pulse as, 'a miserable little weed.' Nevertheless, Florence informed her mother, 'I like Johnson much – not the man of the world & the agreeable companion that Gully is – but far more careful & I could not but admire the pains of the many questions he asked.' The treatment included early rising, exercise, fresh air, relaxation, water treatment, and a well-balanced diet. In the mornings the Nightingales rose even before the other birds were awake for a good hard walk in the pitch dark and the rain. Florence thought morosely of an earlier spa: 'I however am faithful to my first love Malvern. This is so different taking these dreadful Constitutional Walks in the place of the crimson lights and purple shadows, with the most beautiful sunrises in the world, where every look and every breath is a delight.' After their trudge, the Umberslade patients played

* 'Cassandra' referred to herself. In 1852 Florence wrote *Cassandra*, an autobiographical essay attacking family life in which single women were at the will of their parents, married women at the will of their husbands. Thus all women were prevented from pursuing a career.

** The young surgeon was probably Horace Johnson, whose Licentiate of the Society of Apothecaries (LSA) was awarded at Guy's Hospital in 1852.

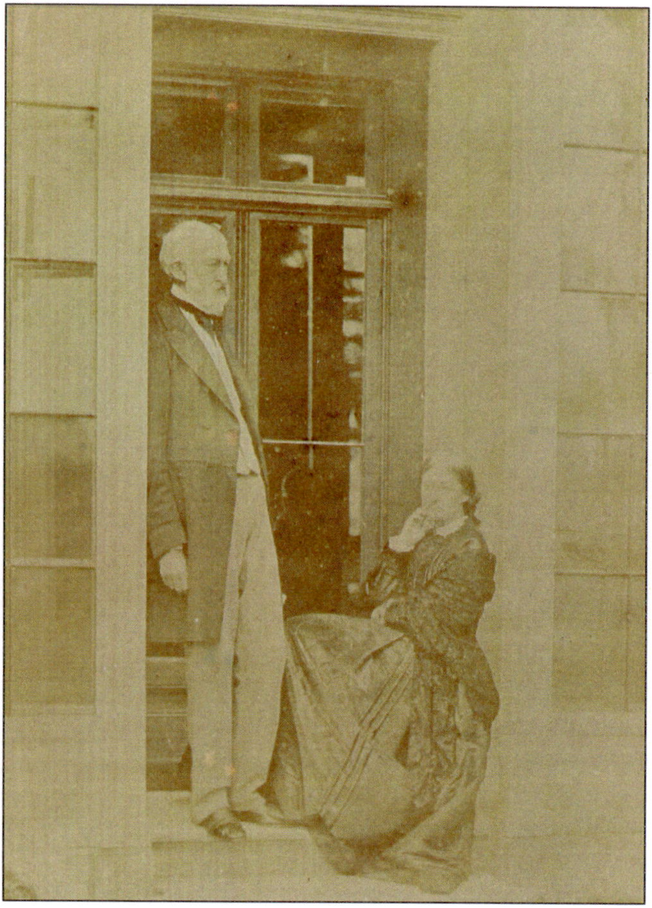

W.E.N and Parthenope at Embley c.1870
Courtesy of Florence Nightingale Trust, London

billiards, followed by breakfast in the dark. Being mid-winter, exercise and relaxation were generally confined indoors, most of the patients playing Blackjack, while the Nightingales played battledore & shuttlecock, 'like two fowls.'

W.E.N was in good spirits and perfectly satisfied with everything, for various reasons. The rooms were good and he and Florence had managed to get adjacent bedrooms; he liked the smallness of the group of patients, and the quietness of the place. He also had an architectural interest in, and appreciation of, the fine Inigo Jones house they were staying in. Umberslade Hall had once belonged to Lord Archer but some years earlier 'the cows were grazing in the dining room with the gilt columns and all the mouldings, now painted out, were then gilt.' But the rooms were once more magnificent and there were plenty of fires. The main thing was that he liked Dr Johnson, as did Florence, who remarked to her cousin, '... I continue to like Dr. Johnson though he is what the world would call vulgate. But he is extraordinarily careful tho' not the genius that Gully is.'

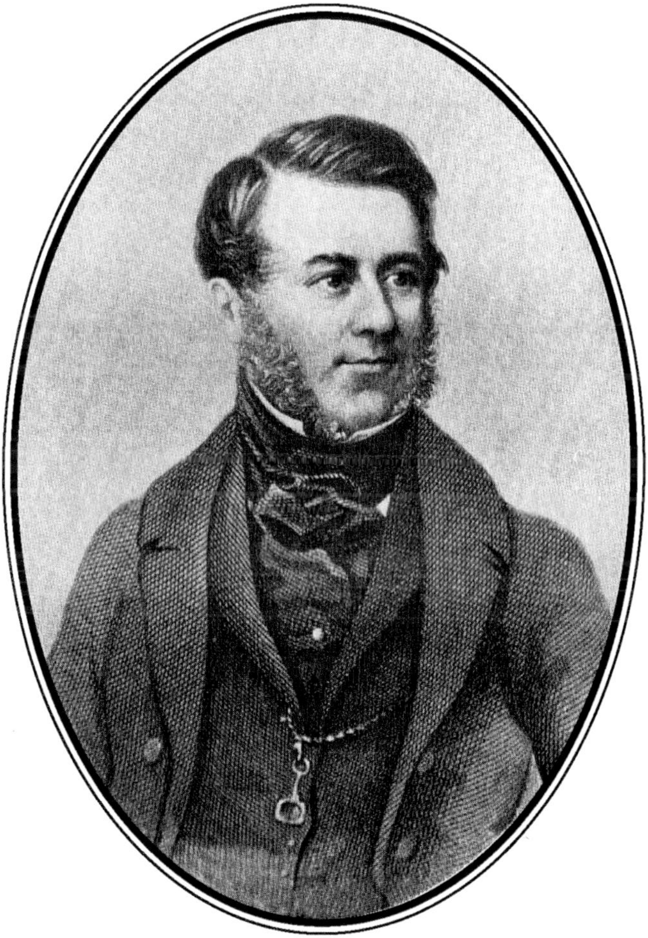

Florence Nightingale liked Dr Edward Johnson, who was careful, clever, practical and liberal, though not a gentleman.

Dr Johnson's natural and successful remedy for curing constipation was a combination of baths, relaxation, exercise, and a balanced diet that included rice, brown bread, meat, fruit, and vegetables. As part of the treatment the patients were weighed every week and Florence was astonished to learn that a boy patient had gained 6lbs weight in one week. Florence considered the water treatment a milder version of Dr Gully's. At first W.E.N had only one dripping sheet and one can douche each day. The 'can douche' was so called because it consisted of two cans of tepid water at 65°F being poured over him. He cheerfully remarked that it would be his restoration. On the Monday after their arrival he began a new treatment of three baths a day. He soldiered on with his intestinal pains which Dr Johnson said would only disappear when the bowels acted - which of course they did. After the first week at Umberslade the bill for board, lodgings and treatment came to £8 3s 0d including fire and candles, which was less than the Nightingales had expected.This seems expensive compared to Harrogate but here she was also paying for treatment. They stayed until the end January.

Florence soon returned to Umberslade Hall. That September Parthe was at Birk Hall, in Ballater, Aberdeenshire, the home of the Queen's physician, Sir James Clark. Writers on the subject have agreed that she was being treated for a mental collapse caused largely by her obsession with her younger, cleverer sister. Parthe's interpretation was that, 'I have been lying on my back, unable to speak or see or understand - but with very little the matter with me but sheer fatigue - for the last three weeks.' It was Florence who travelled to Birk Hall to take Parthe back to Lea Hurst, an agonising journey of several days in which Parthe's condition ranged from sobbing, hearty eating, and being so unwell as to be unable to get into a railway carriage without the physical assistance of a porter. Two months later, in November, Florence went again to Umberslade. '...I am taking the water cure very mildly – only two baths a day - & it always gives me a fillip & my long experience of it makes me feel that I am always the better for it. I felt a good deal knocked up with the Birk Hall story & glad of a little strengthening.'

Chapter VI
The Water Doctors

Dr Edward Johnson (1801-67)

This pioneer of hydropathy in England was born in 1801 in St Germans, Norfolk, and qualified as M.D at the University of Erlangen in Bavaria. He married Frances Amelia and their four sons were all born in Whitechapel.

Dr Johnson spent the winter of 1842-3 studying hydrotherapy at the hands of the master, Vincenz Priessnitz, in the hillside village of Gräfenberg.* On his return to England in 1843 he left his premises in New Burlington Street and took over the hydropathic establishment at Stansteadbury in Hertfordshire. A few months later, in January 1844, one of his patients, Sir Francis Burdett, died. This created great public unease about the Water Cure but Dr Johnson was soon cleared of any blame. By 1847 he had moved to Umberslade Hall in Warwickshire where he treated some notable figures including in 1847 Alfred Tennyson and Black Beauty author Anna Sewell, and W.E.N and Florence Nightingale in 1852. The Nightingales compared Dr Johnson favourably with Dr Gully. W.E.N thought him,'very lavish of his time & conversation, full of advice,' and Florence reassured her mother that, 'He is a good elderly man, not a gentleman like Gully, but clever, practical & liberal.'

In 1854 Dr Edward and Mrs Johnson and their son Dr Walter Johnson left Umberslade Hall and moved to a newly-built hydropathic establishment The Bury [sometimes Malvernbury or Malvern Bury House], at the south end of Abbey Road in Great Malvern. The following year Dr Johnson senior moved to Ellerslie House, a large house a short distance from The Bury, where he treated

* Gräfenberg was formerly in Austrian Silesia but is now in the Czech Republic near its border with Poland.

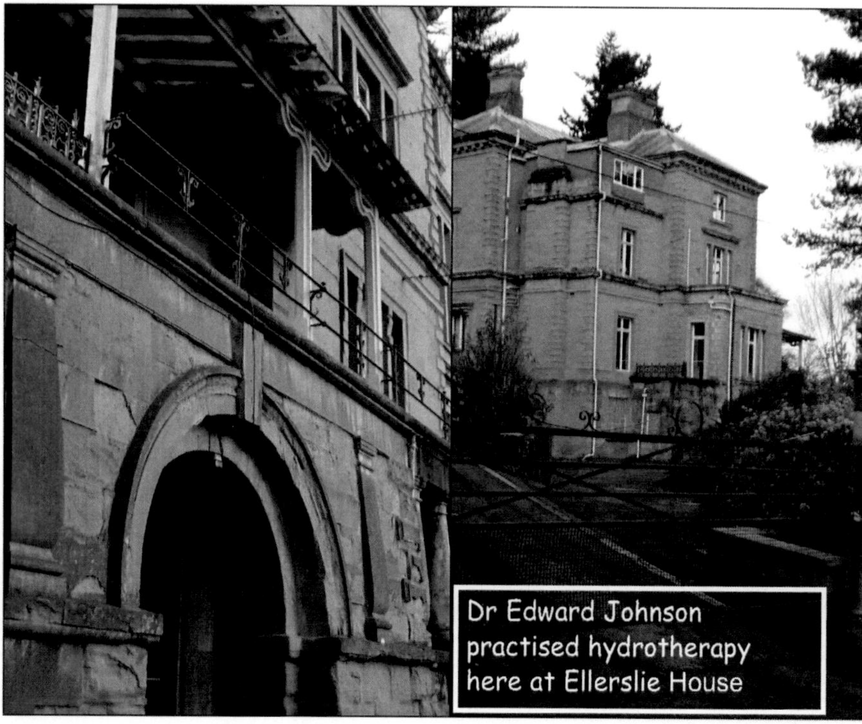

Dr Edward Johnson practised hydrotherapy here at Ellerslie House

his patients. It was essential for the hydropathic establishments to have a constant supply of spring water from the Malvern Hills, since the mains water supply was in such short supply. There was so little of it because there were too few storage tanks so the water ran to waste, and the pipes were described as being about as useful as cardboard. The water was turned on for an hour every two or three days – but the residents were never told which hour it would be switched on. Although Ellerslie House had a 'private supply of the celebrated spring water from the Hill' it clearly was not enough because in June 1856 Dr Edward Johnson applied to the Board of Commissioners for an additional supply of public mains water for hydropathic purposes. The Chairman of the Commissioners, Dr Gully, said that he would write to Dr Johnson about the issue. The following month the Commissioners passed a resolution that the mains water could be used only for domestic purposes unless prior notice was given to the town surveyor. This would have been impossible for

Dr Johnson, who needed a constant supply. Fortunately for Dr Gully, a spring on his property issued 20,000 gallons a day. A year later Dr Edward Johnson retired, perhaps because of the water problem, or through ill-health, and left Ellerslie. After a period of bad health he died at Malvernbury in June 1867 aged 66. He is buried in Malvern cemetery.

Dr Johnson's four sons all became physicians. Howard Frederick was born in August 1825. He gained his M.D at St Andrew's in 1848 and practised in Malvern during the 1860s. It is said that he was at one time connected with a hydro in Finchley which failed. Horace Edward Johnson was born in December 1827. He became M.D at St Andrew's in 1852, LSA Guy's 1852, and LRCP Edinburgh 1859. In the 1850s he ran a hydropathic establishment in a mansion in Oriental Terrace, Brighton. Fortunately no one was injured when, in July 1855, during the Crimean War, the balcony ceiling of an upper apartment collapsed because of the vibrations caused by cannon practise a mile away. William Alfred, born January 1829, wrote *Bedside Letters on Hydropathy* and opened a hydro called Malvern House at Delgany, Co. Wicklow. On 30th April 1861 a man died horribly during a visit to Dr Barter's Turkish Baths in Limerick and within a month Dr W. Johnson had published '*A word to the public on the Turkish Bath*', a critical appraisal of the dangers of such things. His words were skilfully taken to task by Dr T. Rayner, formerly and latterly of Malvern, but at that time proprietor of the Turkish baths in Lower Temple Street, Dublin. In 1864 Dr W. Johnson installed his own Turkish Bath.

Dr Walter Johnson (1824 - 1913)

Dr Walter Johnson was the eldest son of Dr Edward Johnson. Born in London in February 1824 he gained his M.B at the University of London in1847 and assisted his father at his hydropathic practice at Umberslade Hall. In 1854 he and his parents moved to Great Malvern where he was established in a hydropathic practice at The Bury. In January 1858, when Florence Nightingale was staying at his establishment suffering from complete exhaustion, Hilary Bonham

Carter described him as 'very watchful, very thoughtful. He appears to me to be all one could wish for her as a doctor, & you know she thinks highly of him.... She could not have better than here & one thanks God for that.'

In June 1856 Walter's father, Dr Edward Johnson, was denied the use of the mains water to for hydropathic purposes, a decision which almost certainly adversely affected his business. It may also have affected Walter's decision in June 1859 to join the Local Board, a group of twelve commissioners elected in 1851 to run the town. He was appointed to the Finance Committee. Walter married in his 30s and he and his wife, Anna Maria, had four children, all born in Great Malvern. Anna Maria died at Malvernbury at the end of December 1888 aged 54. The following month Dr Johnson advertised his Malvern Hill Cure, which was a prescribed regime of hill walking and healthy diet complemented with a choice of showers, baths and massage. It was a quite changed regime from that of the 1850s and '60s. By 1890 Walter Johnson had, at 66, reached retirement age; he perhaps missed the company of his wife in Malvern, and the Water Cure as he had known it was no more. In December 1890 he and his children left Malvern and moved to London. Dr Walter Johnson, Florence Nightingale's chief hydropathic physician, died in Bayswater in March 1913 leaving an estate valued at £12,658, which is nearly £1 million today.

Doctor James Manby Gully (1808 - 83)

Unlike Dr Edward Johnson, Dr James Manby Gully did not learn his hydropathic skills at the hands of the 'master', Priessnitz. However he was very clever, very well-connected, very charming, very wealthy, and very attractive to women. Born in Jamaica to a wealthy plantation owner, when he was very young he emigrated to Liverpool where he was brought up surrounded by an extended Gully family. In 1829 he took the degree of M.D at Edinburgh and received his Licentiate from the Society of Apothecaries the following year, when he moved to London and established himself as a physician. He married Fanny Court in 1831 and they had four children. Fanny died in 1838 aged 33, shortly after the birth of the fourth child, also Fanny, who died aged two years. Dr Gully remarried disastrously and soon separated from his significantly older spouse.

Perhaps the most dynamic and famous of the country's hydropathic doctors, Dr Gully is remembered for his writing, his skill as a doctor, and his ability to accumulate wealth. For many years he was Chairman of the Malvern Local Board; he was instrumental in the foundation of Malvern's Imperial Hotel and Malvern College, and Manby Road in Malvern is named in his honour. He retired in 1871 and moved to Balham where he died leaving an estate valued at £29,823, which today would be a magnificent £2,238,071.

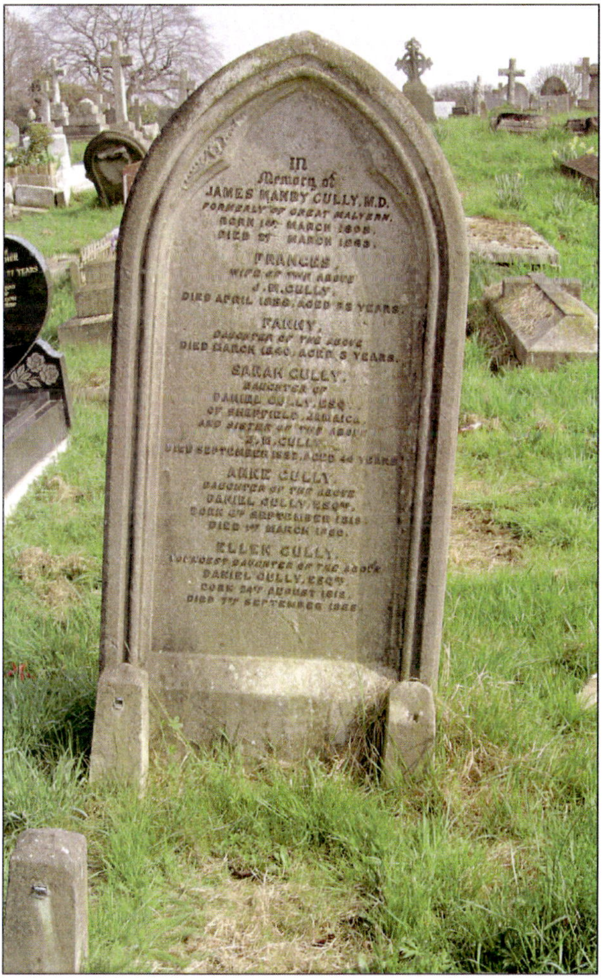
In
Memory of
JAMES MANBY GULLY, M.D.
FORMERLY OF GREAT MALVERN.
FRANCES,
FANNY,
SARAH GULLY,
ANNE GULLY,
ELLEN GULLY,

Dr James Manby Gully was perhaps the most dynamic and famous of the country's hydropathic doctors.

Chapter VII
A State of Complete Exhaustion

Malvern, September 1856

When the Crimean War ended Florence returned quietly and inconspicuously to Lea Hurst, the family home in Derbyshire, on 7th August 1856. She wanted an immediate government-led investigation into the disastrous and preventable loss of life through illness of the soldiers in the Crimea. Ill and exhausted, she was advised by Lord Panmure that it would be better for her to rest, and Sidney Herbert advised her to take note of what his doctor in Carlsbad had advised him: Ni lire, ni écrire, ni réfléchir. [Don't read, don't write, don't think.] Within a month of returning to England she was in Malvern for her health. From *The Glasgow Herald* on 8th September to *Lloyd's Weekly Newspaper* on 21st, a brief item announced that, 'Miss Florence Nightingale is at present sojourning at Malvern, for the purpose of recovering her health.' On 16th September Florence's own local paper, *The Derby Mercury*, reported that, 'Miss Florence Nightingale is now at Malvern and his [sic] under hydropathic treatment.' She was probably resting at Dr Edward Johnson's establishment, Ellerslie House, and while in Malvern may have encountered her former beau Richard Monckton Milnes who was staying with his wife at the Foley Arms Hotel. She could not have been in Malvern above two weeks because on the 16th September she started a two-day journey with her father to Balmoral to meet the Queen and the Prince Consort on the 18th. She visited the Queen again on 4th October and after a healthy break of nearly a month returned south. On 1st November she moved into rooms at the Burlington Hotel in Old Burlington Street with Aunt Mai as her companion, appointment secretary, and kitchen maid.

Malvern, March 1857

Florence endlessly agitated for Parliament to propose a Royal Commission to investigate the conditions of military hospitals and barracks, and the complete reform of the Army Medical Department. Her tenacity resulted in the Queen's endorsement and the government's acquiescence. Although ineligible to sit on the Commission, Florence would be its chief extramural advisor, and give evidence of the results of the Army Medical Corps' inability to save the lives of its soldiers, her 'children'.

The Royal Commission would take a wide range of evidence from many people, mostly who had been in the Crimea, and Florence knew that the Commission's findings would be brutal and horrible. She was working day and night on her 830-page *Notes on Matters affecting the Health, Efficiency and Hospital Administration of the British Army*, in which she relived the ghastly torments of the hospital at Scutari. 'There were very few beds; the poor soldiers were brought down [from the Crimea]with scarcely any clothes, their clothes having been worn off their backs, were placed upon palliasses, and their clothes, at least the remnants of them, full of vermin, taken off their backs and put under the palliasses; no washing had been performed in the hospital, nor the floor washed for six weeks; no washing of linen had been performed; there were no hospital dresses; that there was neither cooking, nor comforts of any kind provided; and as to the whole state of the hospital, it was pestiferous and infectious, the privies being in such a state that nobody could approach the place. This is the description that has been given before this Committee of the state of the hospitals at this time.' Florence wrote on 9th February: 'No one can feel for the army as I do. These people who talk to us have all fed their children on the fat of the land and dressed them in velvet and silk while we have been away. I have had to see my children dressed in a dirty blanket and an old pair of regimental trowsers, and to see them fed on raw salt meat, and nine thousand of my children are lying, from causes which might have been prevented, in their forgotten graves.'

She expected to publish her *Notes* in May 1857 and submit extracts for the Royal Commission, which began its proceedings the same month. It would be a testing time and she needed to be mentally and physically prepared. On 7th March she made it known that she would start ‘active service’ in three months time. She planned to spend the first part of March resting and the remainder of the month in London, apart from a few days visiting Sir John McNeill in Edinburgh. So, early in March, accompanied by Aunt Mai and Buffie*, she went to Malvern. The plan was to rest at Dr Edward Johnson’s water cure establishment, but he was ill in London and had left his establishment in the care of his son Walter. So they drove instead to the Belle Vue Hotel where they learned for the first time about Dr Gully’s Ladies’ Establishment. Florence sent for Dr Gully and had ‘a conference’ with him that evening. She didn’t say anything to Aunt Mai about the consultation except that Gully had spoken out strongly about military mismanagement.

The trio of ladies moved into Holyrood House, which had formerly housed Dr Gully’s male patients. In 1852 he had built a new establishment, Tudor House, adjacent to Holyrood House, and connected the two with an enclosed bridge. He transferred his male patients to Tudor House and installed ladies in Holyrood House. Dr Gully firmly believed that his patients would recover more quickly if living separately, so neither sex was to use the connecting bridge. Hence it became known as - and is still known as - The Bridge of Sighs.

‘Here, we are to breakfast ½ past 8 dine 2. tea 7. We only came after breakfast this morn. & so I have not seen any of our mates. I hope she may let Buffie take her breakfast & tea upstairs. She has a room to herself – Buffie & I another. I like to leave her quite quiet. Buffie goes in & out like a kitten with any message … I hope she will read novels & perhaps sleep. I remember last time at the Water Cure was the only time I ever saw her sleep in the day. She has a comfortable room. She meant to try not to be recognised but Dr Gully sent a letter to her here, directed Miss Nightingale, so of course she is known in the house.’ The news soon leaked to the local newspapers, which announced in mid-March that, ‘Miss Florence Nightingale is at present sojourning at Malvern, at Dr. Gully’s hydropathic establishment.’

* Probably Aunt Mai’s daughter Bertha (1835-1902) who as a baby was known as ‘Buffa’.

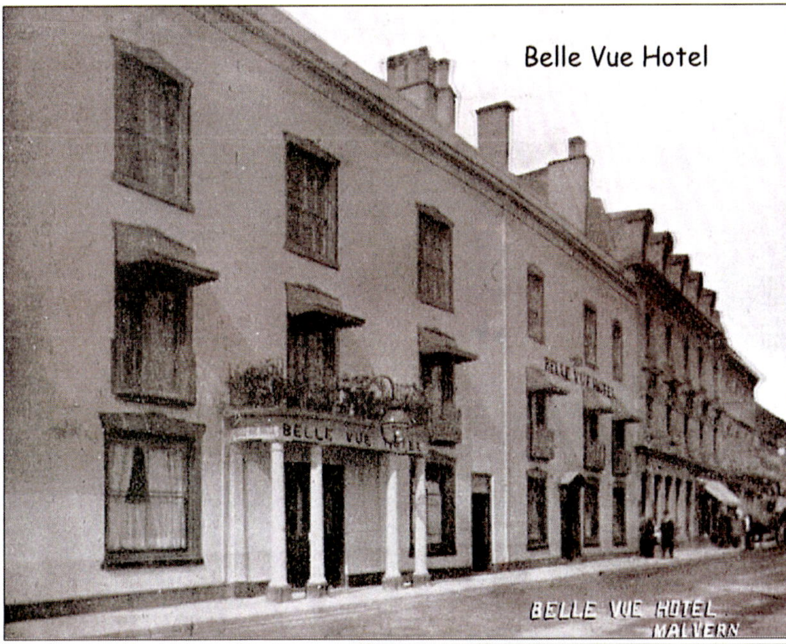

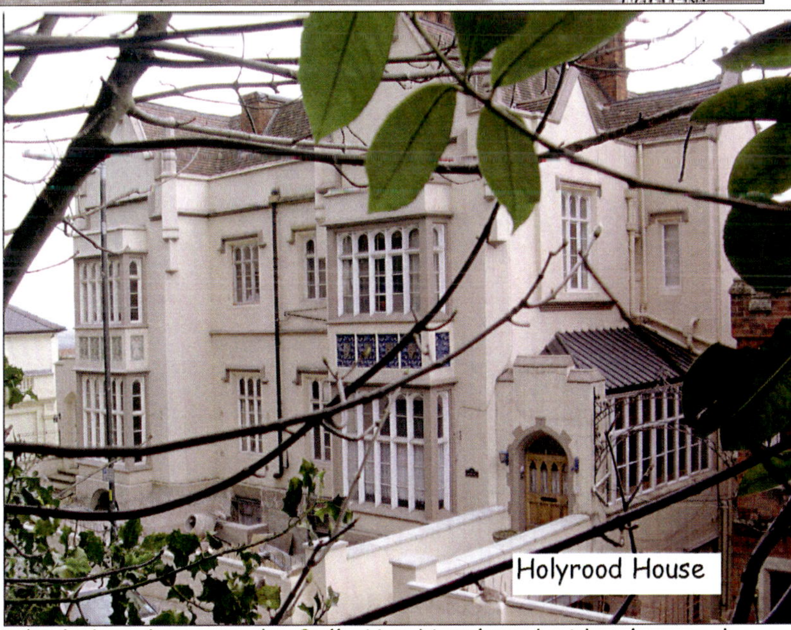

The ladies drove to the Belle Vue Hotel to decide what to do next... and learned for the first time about Dr Gully's Ladies' Establishment, Holyrood House

Dr Gully was very clever, very wealthy, very well-connected, very charming, and very attractive to women.

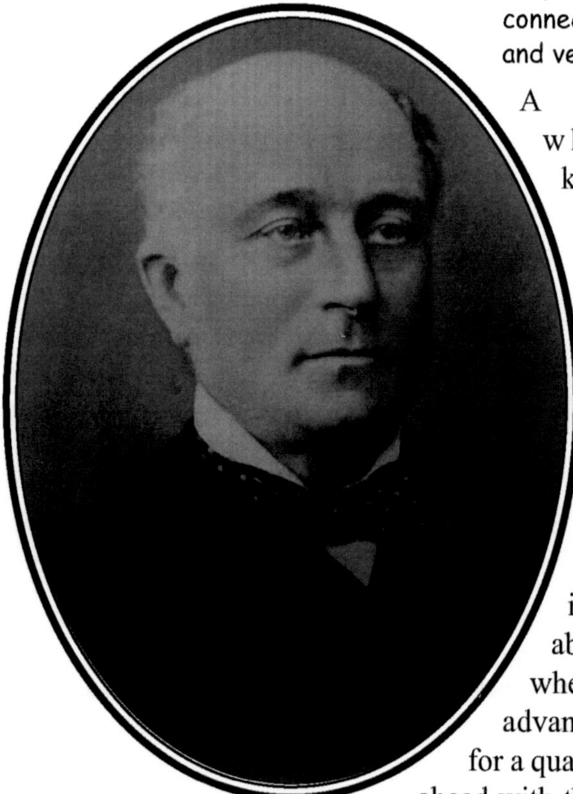

A week later her whereabouts were known round much of the country. 'Miss Florence Nightingale is at present an inmate of the establishment of Dr. Gully, at Holyrood House, Malvern. We understand that her stay at present is likely to be short, but that it is her intention to return in about two months' time, when the season is further advanced, and sojourn here for a quarter of a year - ' Always ahead with the news *The Worcester Herald* affirmed that Florence was not idle, and that: 'This benevolent lady (now staying at Malvern)' had contributed £20 towards the suffering wives and children of the Colchester Camp in Essex.

Malvern, August 1857

Throughout the summer of 1857 Florence laboured day and night trying to resolve the Netley Hospital crisis and preparing her instructions for the Royal Commission into army welfare. In June 1857 Fanny and Parthe offered to go to The Burlington Hotel to look after her. She replied that there was nowhere for them to stay unless she moved out, which was impossible. They still came. She moved out. They acted as receptionists for the constant stream of government visitors, and Fanny wrote a wearisome letter from the Burlington to her husband, telling how they were 'mounting guard over one while she is alone with the other. I am very tired & if it were not for the absolute necessity of our being here to enable her to go on with her most important work should long ago have been back at Embley with you dearest.' Fanny was alarmed that her daughter was working so hard; she had looked out at 1.30 one morning and saw that Florence's light was still on. When she had a word with her, Florence replied, 'When I have work to do which must be finished by a certain time I work great part of the night, sometimes twenty four hours out of 24.'

Parthe related to her father how one day, after a gruelling session preparing her report with Dr John Sutherland, who was advising on medical and sanitary practises, Florence had slipped away for a short rest but within five minutes statistician Dr William Farr arrived 'and she came down immediately & set to work on statistics of the most abstruse kind'. Parthe went on to say how Florence was 'dismally poorly, quite fagged out'. She was as incapable as a five-year-old at looking after herself, unable even to order an egg, and someone had to be there to either put the food into her mouth or stand over her until she had eaten something. But it was not all work for the two carers. They gave breakfasts and dinners, rode in the park, and went out to supper with friends. One night they got back so late that Florence had gone to bed without the supper that they were responsible for providing. The gadding about proved too much and, like Florence, they became ill. Fanny got diarrhoea, and Parthe had a bilious attack and two weeks' worth of headaches, and they consoled each other from comfortable couches. 'It is a scene worthy of Molière,' wrote Florence, 'where two people in tolerable and even perfect health, lie on the sofa all day, doing absolutely nothing and persuading themselves and others that they are the victims of their self-devotion for another who is dying of overwork.' She thought them lazy, overbearing and self-indulgent.

On 21st August Florence fled to Malvern in a state of complete exhaustion. She intended staying at Dr Gully's Ladies' Establishment, where she could be entirely alone. 'She took a sudden resolution yesterday to go to Malvern & nothing would induce her to take any one but George [a footman]', wrote Fanny to W.E.N. 'George is just returned saying that Gully & all other places are so full that there was only a place in Johnson's House quite at the top & there she has taken her weary limbs. It makes us very unhappy to think of her so forlorn and comfortless.' Water Cure patients would normally book accommodation in advance to avoid this situation, which is an indication of the urgency of Florence's need to escape.

On 25th August she wrote to her mother from Bury House, Great Malvern. 'Dearest Mother.... I am resting in the entire quiet here & shall not move this week. I am glad to be alone.' She may have wanted to be alone, but her whereabouts was no secret.

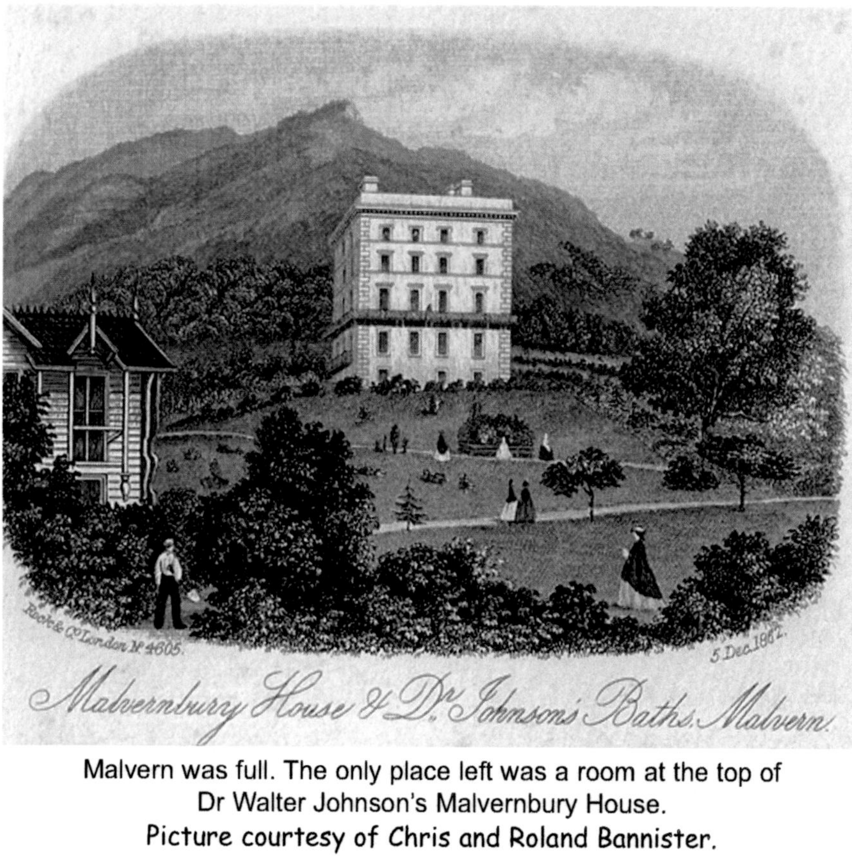
Rock & Co London No 4605.
5 Dec 1862.
Malvernbury House & Dr Johnson's Baths, Malvern.

Malvern was full. The only place left was a room at the top of Dr Walter Johnson's Malvernbury House.
Picture courtesy of Chris and Roland Bannister.

On 9th September *The Derby Mercury* mentioned to the world the whereabouts of the nation's favourite heroine. *The Worcester Herald* carried the same story on 12th September 1857:

> 'MISS NIGHTINGALE – This estimable lady is staying at
> Great Malvern for the benefit of the cold water cure, at
> Dr. Walter Johnson's hydropathic establishment.'

Eventually Florence was joined by Aunt Mai, who allowed in only the visitors Flo wished to see and who kept the family informed of her condition. She was very unwell. When W.E.N visited he was horrified by the severity of his younger daughter's condition. Her distress was obvious from her laboured breathing; she was unable to eat if at all agitated, and she consequently suffered sleepless nights. 'Her days may be numbered,' he wrote to Fanny. 'Tis a sad tale. I'm not able to say any more. Adieu....'

In September 1857 Parthe wrote to Madame Mohl [formerly Mary Clarke], 'The accounts of F. have been very anxious. Aunt Mai says she does not sleep above two hours in the night, and continues most feverish and feeble, and cannot eat. She never left that room where you saw her, was scarcely off her sofa for a month. Now she goes down for half an hour into a parlour, to do business with a Commissioner who has been there to see her... both doctors say there is no disease, that it is only entire exhaustion of every organ from overwork, and that rest alone will restore her... She has two "packs" a day; this is all the water-curing; it seems to bring down the pulse, and she lies at that open window the chief part of the day, not reading or writing, only just still. She cannot be better anywhere, no one can get at her; Aunt Mai is a dragon, and the Commissioner is the only person who has seen her. Aunt Mai says, "I cannot disguise to myself that she is in a very precarious state."'

The Commissioner was Dr John Sutherland. At Parthe's instigation he had written to Florence, and in reply she explained to him how, as soon as she had arrived in Malvern, she was put on a sofa and told not to move or take any solid food at all until her pulse came down.

She added that after any walk or drive she sat up all night with palpitations, and felt sick at the sight of any animal food. She humorously but wryly enquired whether he thought her like one of Byron's young ladies as it was he, she thought, who had made small appetites fashionable. Although she was weak in body, she was strong in determination, and begged him to go to Malvern to discuss her work. He resisted the invitation, and wrote two letters to her at the end of August begging her to stop work and recover her health. She did not stop work. He went to Malvern. Upon his arrival on 14th September he took lodgings at the Abbey boarding house in Abbey Road where Aunt Mai was also staying. He also found Florence in a dreadful state. She was too weak to leave the sofa during the day and could not sleep more than two hours at night. Her pulse raced, and for this she was given two cold water packs each day. Then the tables turned; he became ill, and Florence was obliged to send his wife a progress report of the 'sick baby'. Another visitor to Malvern at that time was her dear friend Richard Monckton Milnes. She had turned down his offer of marriage in 1849 but they had remained firm friends and he was a trustee of the Nightingale Fund, which was officially launched in November 1855. He left Malvern for Carmarthen at the end of September and Florence, Aunt Mai and Dr Sutherland at the beginning of October.

Florence Nightingale later received an account dated 31 Oct 1857 from Dr Walter Johnson at Malvern Bury House, for ten days' treatment.*

	£	s	d
Treatment 10 days	6	0	0
Fires		7	6
Candles		1	6
Servant 1 day		3	0
Total	6	12	0

* Found in Cope, Zachary, *Florence Nightingale and the Doctors*, p133

Malvern Bury House operated as an 'ordinary', where a fixed daily or weekly rate was charged, in this case twelve shillings a day [four guineas a week] for board and treatment. Dr Johnson probably operated a sliding scale of charges, in line with the other three main hydropathic establishments. Doctors Wilson and Gully charged from two to six guineas per week depending on the rank of the patient, type of accommodation required and extent of treatment. According to one young male patient, Dr Grindrod's 'ordinary terms to out patients is 2 guineas a week.... For the 14 weeks he charged Aunt Elizabeth £5 & for me £7. The difference I suppose because I was of some trade & she a servant.' Like Malvernbury, most lodgings also made 'extraordinary' charges for heating, lighting, and domestic help. Was Florence Nightingale's visit expensive? How affordable was this to the average person in 1857? The average weekly earnings of a Worcestershire agricultural labourer in 1860, was just ten shillings, so ten days at Dr Johnson's was prohibitively expensive.Using the Retail Price Index, £6 12 0d is today worth £438.31.

Florence's treatment was followed by several weeks of convalescence. Four pieces of evidence suggest that she did not convalesce at Dr Johnson's but at Dr Gully's, where she had originally intended to go. Firstly is the bill from Dr Johnson for only ten days' treatment, which would have been from 21st to 30th August. Secondly, on 25th August she had written to her mother from Bury House that she was resting, '& shall not move this week'. This suggests that she had intentions of moving out of Johnson's, perhaps the following week. Thirdly, in his correspondence to her, Dr Sutherland had urged,'... Please don't gull Dr. Gully, but do eat and drink and don't think.' He is unlikely to have said this if she were staying at Dr Johnson's. Fourthly, an undated letter from Aunt Mai, recipient unknown but probably Fanny, suggests that she and Sam should go to Malvern to be with Florence so that Sam could consult Dr Gully about his condition. On the other hand, several newspapers in mid-September had reported that Florence was staying at Dr Johnson's but the newspapers were often late with their news.

Chapter VIII
Miss Nightingale's Health

Florence Nightingale arrived in Balaklava, Crimea, on 3rd May 1855. Immediately she set about visiting the various English hospitals there. She was out for hours each day in wet, chilly weather and barely had time to eat. She did not always appear in the best of health. On 13th May, the day after her 35th birthday, she became seriously ill and was immediately take by stretcher to the Castle Hospital on the Genoese Heights. From there she could hear 'the everlasting report of the cannon' at Sebastopol.

Mrs Eliza Roberts, one of the Scutari nurses, who had accompanied Florence to the Crimea as her personal nurse, announced that Florence was dangerously ill with the worst form of Crimean fever. The attending doctor, Dr Anderson, said she was suffering from the worst attack of fever he had ever seen. The extrovert and indispensable Reform Club chef Alexis Soyer (1809-58) told Lord Raglan 'of her imprudence in visiting a patient at Dr Henderson's [sic], who had been attacked by the worst form of Crimean fever; also, of her remaining out so late, and not taking any refreshment.' She was not expected to live. Her personal physician, Dr Sutherland, reported that she was having all the attention she needed and that she should be left in peace with no visitors except the doctors and Mrs Roberts. Not even Charles Bracebridge, who had also travelled with them, was allowed access. Her illness caused palpitations, insomnia, spinal pain, loss of appetite, nausea, racing pulse, depression, undulating fever, delirium, and extreme mental and physical exhaustion. She was so weak she could not feed herself, even if she had an appetite; she became emaciated, pale, and debilitated. After three weeks she was out of danger and only well enough to return by ship to Scutari on 5th June for several weeks' recuperation. Her Crimean illness was diagnosed in 1995 by David Young, a former principal scientist at the

Wellcome Institute in London, as the symptoms of brucellosis, known as 'undulant fever' because of its intermittent recurrences, sometimes many years apart. Florence probably caught it through consuming unpasteurized milk and contaminated cheese. The illness is exacerbated by stress.

When she arrived at Malvern in 1857 Florence was suffering several symptoms of Crimean Fever: insomnia, loss of appetite, racing pulse, weakness, physical exhaustion, palpitations, and nausea. This was probably accompanied by stress, which can cause both physical and emotional health problems, characterised by her tiredness and insomnia, digestive problems, raised heart rate, and disturbed eating patterns. There were many reasons for her stressed condition, not least being the overpowering and irritating intrusion of her mother and sister into her London life; who expected her to do, to be, and to think exactly as they demanded. She was also mentally and physically exhausted. Following her slow recovery from fever during the summer of 1855, she worked through the cold winter while suffering bouts of rheumatism and sciatica, dysentery, earache and laryngitis. At the end of the war she had accounts and reports to complete and was one of the last to return to England. When she finally arrived home her immediate aim was not to rest but to secure the reform of the health administration of the British army.

Florence may also have been suffering from post traumatic stress disorder [PTSD], which is characterised by irritability and outbursts of anger. Also, difficulty in sleeping, estrangement from other people and activities, and believing ones life will not last much longer - which she did for many post-War years. One example occurred in 1857 when, believing she was close to death, she wrote to Sidney Herbert, 'I am sorry not to stay alive to do the "*Nurses*". But I can't help it...' PTSD might have been caused by the terrible events at Scutari; by her helplessness at watching soldiers (whom she referred to as her children) dying of disease and wounds because of her inability at first to do little to improve their chances. She knew that at her badly-equipped, ill-ventilated, half-ruinous hospital at Scutari, the death rate was far higher than in the military hospitals in the Crimea; that the poor drainage and sanitation; the inadequate ventilation, lavatories and washing installations, and the insufficient food supply and cooking facilities, meant that sick or wounded soldiers sent to her hospital stood almost no chance of survival. 'Oh my poor men who endured so patiently, I feel I have been such a bad mother to you, to come home and leave you lying in your Crimean grave 73 per cent in 8 Regt during 6 months from disease alone,' she had written in a note at the end of 1856. When she returned home from the East she was 'haunted by thoughts of the 'living skeletons' of that dreadful first winter; men, ulcerated and covered with vermin, who wrapped their heads in their blankets, and died without uttering a word.... Almost a decade after the war, she was to look back and shudder at the memory of the 'slaughter houses' of Scutari. It was like a 'horrid spectre' that she was afraid of conjuring up from the dark corners of her mind, where it was ever present, waiting to spring out on her.'

She may also have been suffering from delayed Shell Shock, a term used in the Great War to describe the psychological trauma of men fighting on the front line. Symptoms included insomnia, palpitations and depression. Shell Shock is not necessarily caused by loud noises, as the term implies, but in this case, 'The cannon of Sebastopol made a fearful noise', which Florence would have been able to hear from her hospital bed at Balaklava. On 2nd Oct 1857 Aunt Mai informed Florence's family 'that her state of nerves makes her hear sounds at a distance quite beyond hearing when she is well, & that when a cart went along at Malvern ... it was the feeling of an earthquake.' It seems that there may have been more than one cause of Florence's complete prostration in 1857.

Chapter IX
Propped up by Pillows

Malvern, December 1857 to March 1858

On 12th December 1857 *The Worcester Herald* trumpeted: 'Miss Nightingale is at Vienna, and is treated with great distinction. She frequently visits the hospitals'. Messages flooded in to Burlington Street congratulating Florence on her recovered health, and since she was better people wanted, and expected, to visit her. Two weeks after running the story the paper admitted getting the story wrong; that since her arrival back in England from the Crimean War Florence Nightingale had not left the country and 'we regret to hear that her health still continues much impaired by her exertions on behalf of our sick and wounded soldiers during the late war.' The footman, John Bratby, and his wife Mary, were instructed to say, upon enquiry, that their mistress was 'much the same'.

Within a few weeks of leaving Malvern in October, Florence had had a relapse and in November she made her will. By December she was seriously ill, panting for breath, sleepless, and not eating. Her physician, Dr Williams, did not think her life was in danger, and thought that she would live for years, but he questioned for how much longer she might be able to work. Aunt Mai was so anxious that she went to Malvern where she managed a hurried interview with Dr Johnson to get his opinion of Florence's condition. He wrote his thoughts to Aunt Mai, who was upset at 'the anxious tenor of his letter'. Dr Williams forbade Florence to go to Malvern because he did not think she had the strength to make the journey. He prescribed egg beaten up with wine and arrowroot, an easily digestible invalid's diet that had been widely prescribed for the sick Scutari soldiers. Parthe, herself unwell and being treated by Sir James Clark, was very disappointed at Dr Williams' decision. Arthur Clough prepared his

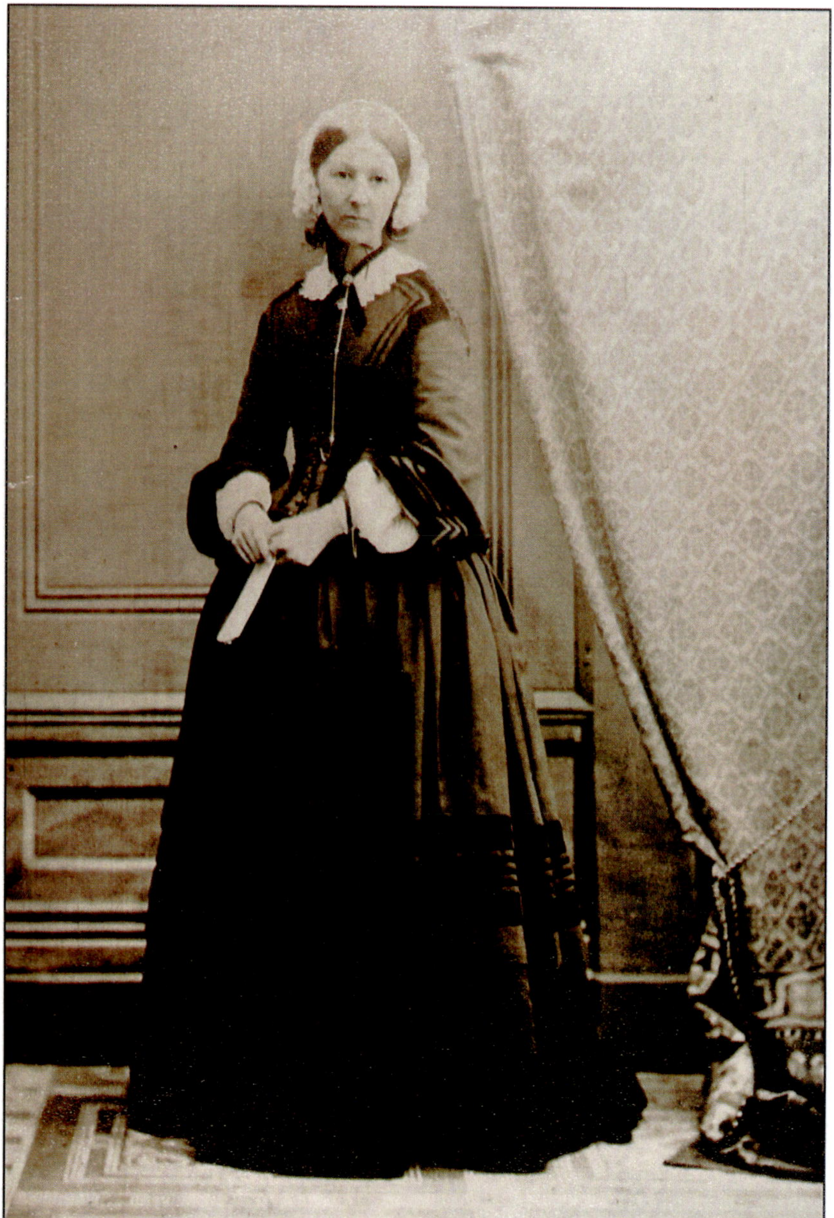

This photograph by Goodman shows Florence c.1857 looking thin, with her formerly long chestnut locks cropped short. Photograph courtesy Florence Nightingale Trust, London.

house, Combe Hurst on Kingston Hill, in case she decided to go there, but Florence believed that 'her much tried experience of Malvern' would be the best place for her if her health was to improve, and that is where, she confided in Arthur Clough, that against doctor's orders she had decided to go. John Bratby got the carriages ready. He and his wife Mary, and Arthur Clough, escorted Florence to Malvern so that if the journey proved too much they could help her find accommodation in Worcester before continuing to Malvern. As it happened, Aunt Mai was right in thinking that Florence would find it less fatiguing to go straight to Malvern. On arrival at Malvern the Bratbys were immediately to leave for Embley and give a report of Florence's progress to her parents.

Aunt Mai asked her niece Hilary [Bonham Carter] to return to Malvern where she had just been for 'the watering' to recover from a head ailment. Hilary particularly liked Malvern because, as a keen painter, she could find life models there. Aunt Mai instructed Hilary to book in to Roslin House in the Southfields [now College Road] and be on hand to assist Florence wherever necessary and write constant reports to the family. Florence was not to be told of this arrangement because she would worry that Hilary was giving up too much time for her and not getting on with her painting. So it was agreed that Hilary would tell Florence that she was going there for her own health. This was true, because she thought a little more treatment for her head would be beneficial, and because it was the ideal place to get on with some painting. She was instructed not to be in a hurry to get to Malvern because Florence always had a few days there, or even a week, completely on her own. Roslin House was not ideal. It had good, large, east-facing rooms but it was cold, and the sitting rooms were small. Hilary and Aunt Mai ignored these drawbacks, and stayed there because it was near Dr Johnson's and they liked the two respectable and obliging ladies who ran it. Of the other accommodation the Abbey lodging house was recommended, though W.E.N objected to staying there because the new church clock was such a noisy nuisance at night, with its striking every quarter hour.

On Tuesday 29th December 1857 Florence left London once more for Malvern, arriving at Dr Walter Johnson's in the evening. She was there for five days before Hilary saw her on the Saturday morning, and she seemed no worse for the strenuous journey. By then the severest exhaustion had passed and there had been no relapse. Florence was so glad to be in Malvern, and at The Bury she had two rooms with their own little corridor. The bedroom was large and pleasant and she spent most of the day lying in a comfortable bed with a sprung mattress. Hilary read all the letters that arrived but Florence

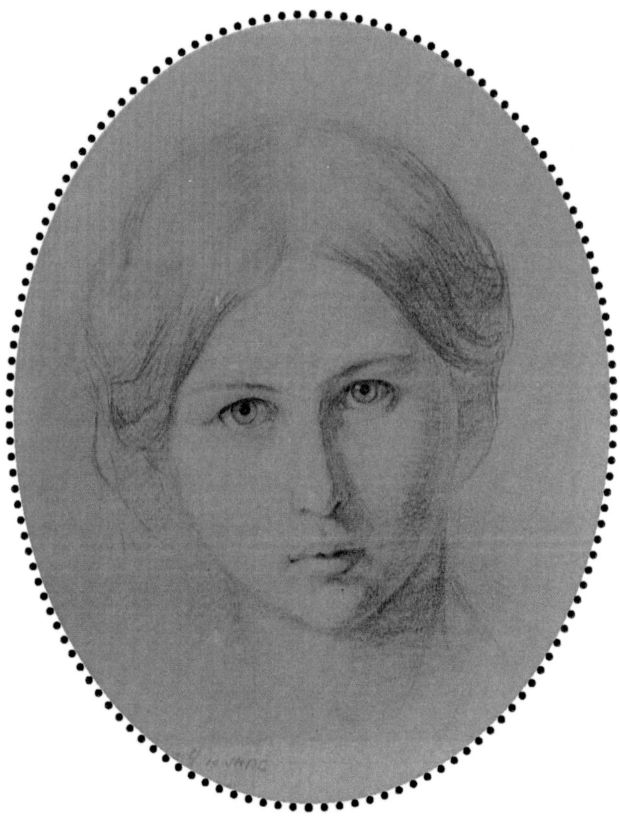

Hilary Bonham Carter returned to Malvern to look after her cousin, Florence Nightingale, who was seriously ill.
Picture courtesy Florence Nightingale Museum Trust, London.

Hilary and Aunt Mai moved into Roslin House, which was conveniently close to Malvernbury.

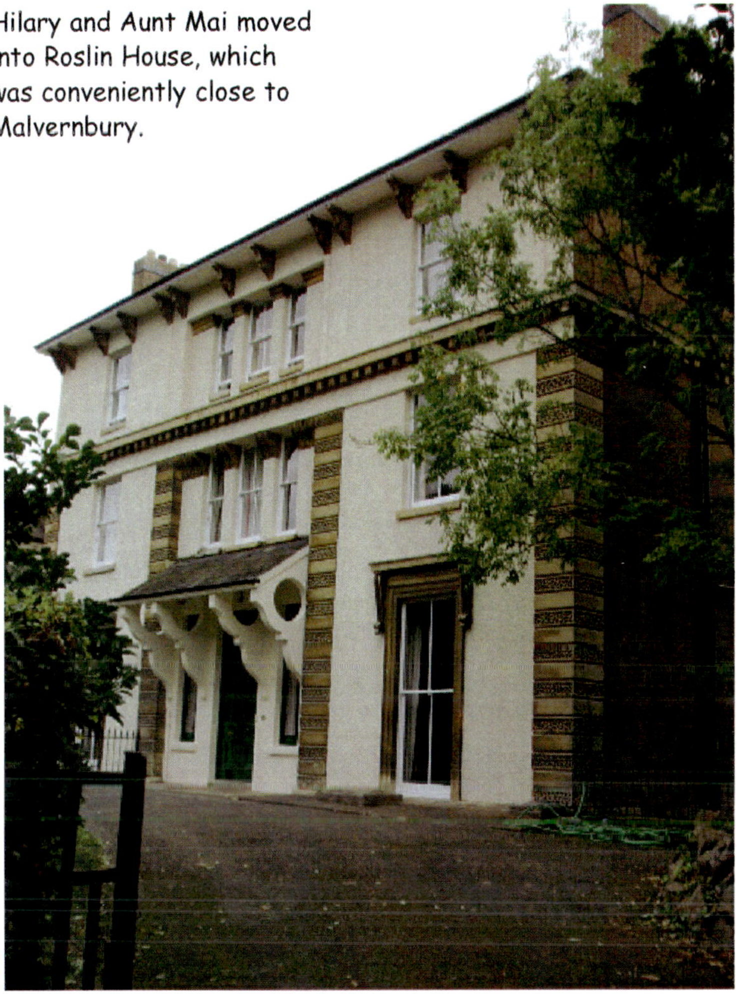

found it much too tiring to write lying down so dictated her few replies to Hilary. Every afternoon she went into the smaller room, which caught the midday sun, and there for two or three hours she lay propped up by pillows on the sofa with the windows open, enjoying the pure air. Malvern was surprisingly warm for the time of year, much warmer than down below in the Severn valley. Hilary had seen – or rather heard – a waggoner coming up the road who told her it was a completely different world up in town than down in the valley, where the frost was so hard that it could support the weight of a horse.

Florence was well looked after by two 'old ladies', 35-year-old Charlotte Packer and 52-year-old Mary Jenkins, the two resident bathwomen at Dr Johnson's. Florence already knew Mary, who had been working for Dr Edward Johnson at Umberslade Hall when she and W.E.N visited in 1852, and had come with Dr Johnson to Malvern. Mary told Hilary, 'You know, Ma'am she doesn't mind us no more than two little cats running about'.

About a week after Florence arrived Hilary wrote to Aunt Mai asking her to send a water bed that had belonged to Fanny, and which Hilary thought would be useful to Florence. Also to send a flannel jacket which would be snug when she was sitting up in bed. In the end Hilary bought a water mattress in town but Florence didn't use it because she found her new elastic hair mattress was just right. Hilary reported that Mary, the bathwoman, had said that she thought Florence showed signs of improvement but it was slow and not much. Dr Johnson was doing all he could to help, and was anxious that she should have complete rest.There were only a few patients in the house but it was not built for quiet so he installed a baize door to shut her apartment off from the rest of the house. He ensured that she was saved from any and every exertion or disturbance, particularly caused by seeing people, hoping that any strength she had was saved to do the things she wanted to do, notably 'the work to which she has been called'. Her mother had sent some game to Lady Coltmore in Malvern, who had cooked the pheasant and turned it into tasty little morsels, and made the hare into soup. Dr Johnson made sure Florence was taken a tasty little morsel every hour from 6am until 8pm, but her strength and appetite had deserted her and she ate very little, although she never left the food completely untouched.

Florence wrote to her mother on 6th January 1858. 'To my dearest Mother I apply for ease and for help in my present pressing and difficult circumstances... I am obliged now to restrict myself to one companion or, rather, I should say that companionships can be no more for me, while my work remains unfinished....' She then put off either her mother or her sister from being that 'one companion',

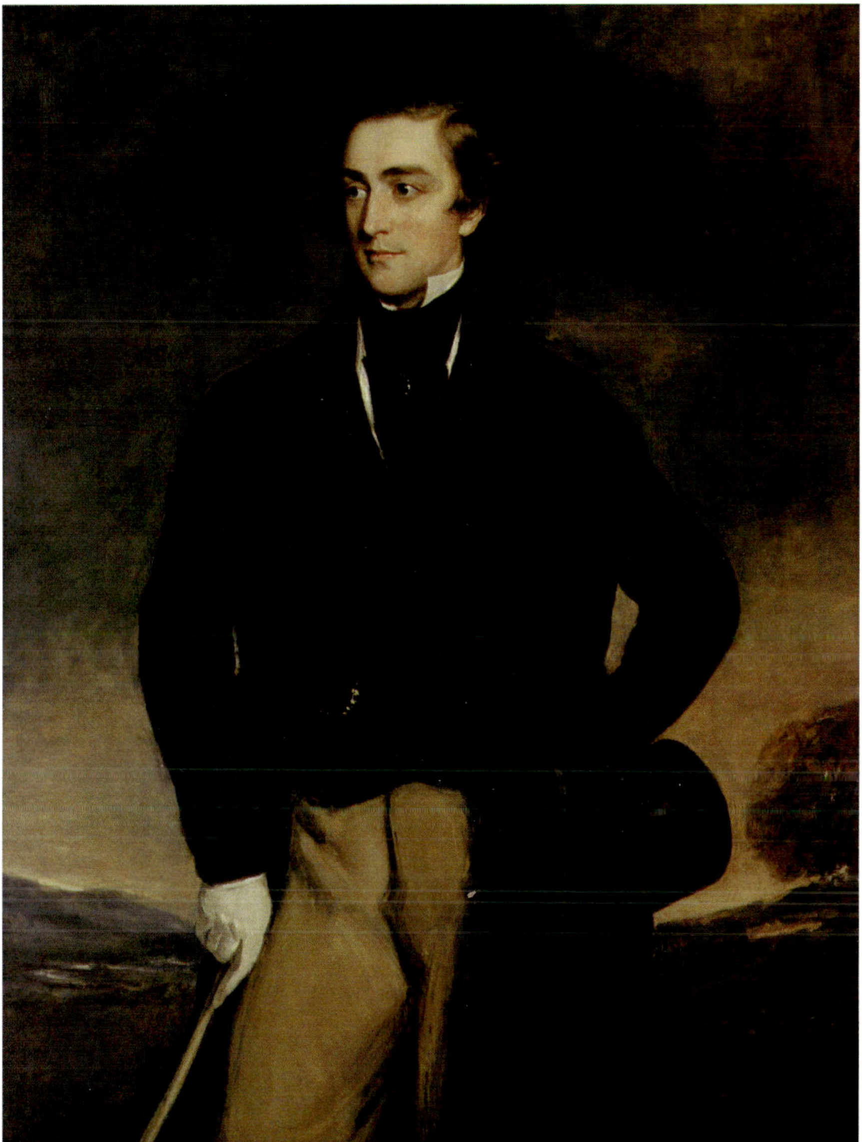

Sidney Herbert, 1st Baron Herbert of Lea, by Sir Francis Grant. Oil on canvas, 1847. National Portrait Gallery, London.
Sidney Herbert was a perfect English gentleman and Florence Nightingale's most important friend. She could not have achieved her ambitions without his help.

saying that if it were either of them she would become anxious about their health, and that she would be putting them through the 'sort of life I am compelled to require'. Her remaining physical and mental power she would use 'to rescue the children committed to me from death, from disease, from immorality.' To this end Dr Sutherland spent many hours with her on her report for the Royal Commission, but she was also corresponding with Sidney Herbert about the catastrophe surrounding the ill-conceived plans for Netley Hospital. She also started to take control of her life in London. She had found her mother and sister more pressure than help in London, so when her father offered to find accommodation there for the three of them she politely turned his offer down and said she would ask Aunt Mai to come and help her with her work. Selena Bracebridge also offered to find accommodation in London, but Flo reiterated that Aunt Mai and Uncle Sam would do that for her.

Florence received a constant stream of visitors. Dr Sutherland was in Malvern by mid-January; Aunt Mai's daughter Beatrice was returned to Malvern while Mai's husband Sam and another daughter, Bertha, came from Weymouth on 17th. Sidney Herbert was expected the following day, and although Florence had been 'very poorly' and not up for several days she would go downstairs to see him when he arrived. On Monday 25th January Hilary wrote to her Aunt Fanny and Uncle W.EN to say there was little day-to-day change in Florence's condition. She had a basic daily routine, but any further exertion would lead to more exhaustion. She also told Uncle W.E.N that Florence hoped he would visit either on the Thursday, Friday or Saturday that week. He arrived on the Thursday and immediately went to see Florence. She was lying on a sofa and had been forbidden to leave it – not even to go into the next room. Despite her physical weakness her voice and manner were strong about the subjects most on her mind. In particular was the reorganisation of the Indian army and the preparation of comparative sketches of civil and military hospitals in Paris and London, those in Paris being of a much higher standard than those in London. W.E.N did not think that Parthe would be allowed to visit because it would cause Florence too much 'emotional agitation' and felt that the 'least excitement may realise Johnson's forebodings.'

Florence's condition undulated. In early February her future brother-in-law, Sir Harry Verney, visited to discuss hospital engineering with her. In mid-February W.E.N received a letter from Hilary suggesting that Florence's life was in danger. That was the month that the long-awaited Royal Commission on the Health of the Army Report was published. On 10th March Sir Harry Verney commented that Florence was so occupied that he had barely seen her for more than five minutes but hoped that her health improved. Six days later he reported that Dr Sutherland was sure that Florence was not suffering from any organic disease. Aunt Mai had at one time anticipated that Florence would leave Malvern at the end of the first week in February, but it was towards the end of March that she was finally well enough to return home to London.

Malvern, August 1858

The *Derby Mercury* of 11th August 1858 reported that, 'MISS NIGHTINGALE'S HEALTH is such that she has again been obliged to resort to Malvern for the water cure.' The newspaper was local to Lea Hurst, so probably the first to pick up the story, which was repeated in newspapers throughout the country. By then Florence had been in Malvern for almost two weeks. After her usual few days of solitude Aunt Mai, Uncle Sam and one of their daughters, Aunt Joanna Bonham Carter with her daughter Hilary and one of her sisters, and Dr and Mrs Sutherland, all arrived at Roslin House. Florence stayed for two months, in the hope of as complete a rest and recovery as possible. Then, escorted by Aunt Mai, she arrived back in London on 1st October. According to the *Malvern News*, the remainder of the entourage stayed for another couple of weeks.

Malvern, January 1859 and March 1859

At the beginning of 1859 Florence revisited Malvern, the health of the army very much on her mind. On 7th and 8th January she wrote letters to Sir John McNeill about officers' responsibility for the health of their troops. She wrote to Sir John Richardson about the functions of Medical Inspection Officers in the army and navy and she dropped a line to Harriet Martineau, encouraging her to write articles in the newspapers about the health of the army and bring the crisis to public attention. On 9th February she wrote to Harriet Martineau of her imminent return to London. This was not to be.

Nearly a month later, on 4th March 1859 *The London Daily News* reported that, 'Miss Florence Nightingale is now staying at Malvern, at the water establishment of Dr Johnson.' *The Leeds Mercury* ran the same story the following day. As May crossed into June countless local newspapers were running another story: that Miss Florence Nightingale had entered a Roman Catholic convent at Gorey, County Wexford. Within days, countless numbers of local newspapers were admitting that the story, despite being obtained 'on good authority', was not true. Worse than that, and completely true, was that her health was in 'a most precarious state'.

Her health continued to cause alarm. In February 1860, local newspapers reported that, 'We regret to learn that a still greater change for the worse has taken place in the health of Miss Florence Nightingale than was even lately announced when great fears were entertained. She has left Hampstead for London in consequence.' A year later she was still unwell. 'MISS NIGHTINGALE'S HEALTH – We regret to learn from yesterday's *Times*, upon "undoubted authority" that the report recently circulated by several journals of the improvement in Miss Nightingale's health is entirely without foundation. Her malady, far from being alleviated, increases upon her, and her state, which confines her entirely to her apartment, is one of great exhaustion and severe suffering.' And later in 1861, 'ILLNESS OF FLORENCE NIGHTINGALE - A letter from Florence Nightingale has been published in which she says, "There is no prospect but of my health becoming ever worse and worse till the hour of my release."' In August that year Aunt Mai reported to Fanny that Florence seemed 'very much worse, her face & hands so swollen..' and on Christmas Eve she suffered severe spinal pain. Throughout the

1860s and 1870s she had recurring bouts of nausea, fainting, and weakness. The worst symptoms did not decrease until the early 1880s.

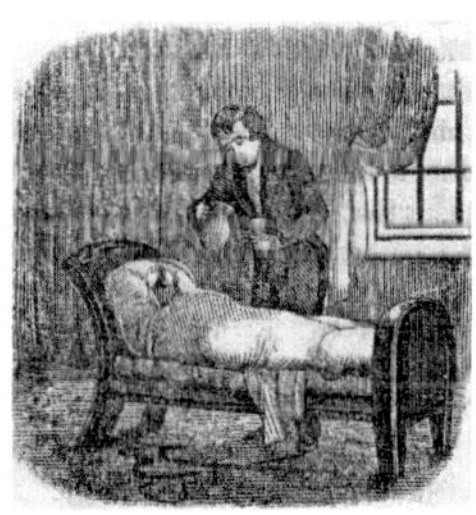

Chapter X
An End to the Misery

Florence Nightingale endorses the Water Cure

In 1854 Florence's cousin Blanche married Arthur Hugh Clough. He had a close working relationship with Florence and she was extremely fond of him. In 1859 a succession of illnesses and the pressure of work made him depressed and ill. In September 1860 he told Florence that he was thinking seriously of visiting Malvern. She would have endorsed his choice because, following her own treatment, she had changed her earlier opinion that the water cure was a novel amusement for bored, wealthy hypochondriacs with plenty of time on their hands.

Her opinion of the Water Cure at this time is revealed in a letter of 1860 to Edwin Chadwick. She wrote, ' ... I should not be here were it not for Malvern. In August 1857, after my work at the Royal Sanitary Commission, and after four weeks of anxiety and exertion, I was told that my life was not worth 24 hours purchase – and I knew it too. I owe three years of ... life to the water-cure at Malvern.' Chadwick suspected that the water cure was just another quackery but she warned, 'don't disparage the wet sheet packing - I know it has saved many lives in fever. I am sure it saved mine.' We can be in no doubt that the woman we admire more than any other in the world of health reform had recovered her own health through hydropathy. She had seen the same result many times in others. She understood how and why hydropathy worked; had studied and approved its merits and application, had asked dozens of questions, and been satisfied with the answers.

The Water Cure of course is not a cure-all. In November 1860 Clough visited Malvern and, accompanied by his wife Blanche, her parents Aunt Mai and Uncle Sam, and her sisters Bertha and Beatrice, he took Charleforde, a large house in Priory Road. Within a year he was dead.

Malvern, 1867

Florence did not visit Lea Hurst between 1858 and 1867, Embley between 1859 and 1866, or Malvern between 1859 and 1866. She confined herself to barracks but by the end of 1866 she needed to get away. She noted how she, '...broke up all at once and fled to Malvern on December 26th with a little cat'. She stayed for nine days, reading nothing and seeing no one. Dr Sutherland was the only person who knew where she was, and that was at The Bury with Dr Walter Johnson. She wrote to her mother on 11th January thanking her for a food hamper and describing the benefits of being in Malvern. 'As for

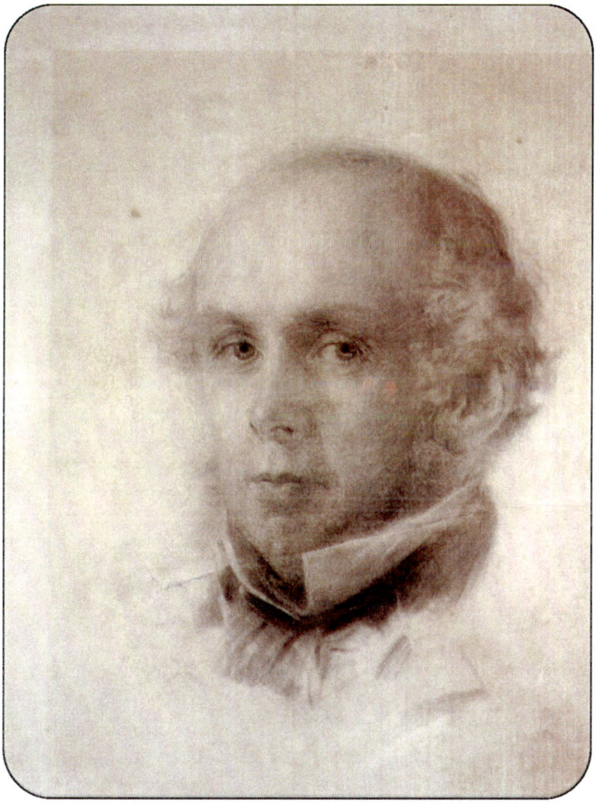

Arthur Hugh Clough by Samuel Rowse, chalk, 1860
National Portrait Gallery, London
Arthur Clough was devoted to Florence's service. He corrected her proofs, posted her parcels and attended to her travel arrangements.

my coming here: it certainly has answered. Nothing else would have broken off the perpetual grind stone, the tread wheel of my life in London but my total disappearance. People (not government people) had got into the habit of sending me their business at all hours... I have been interrupted thus three times in one page in a letter to Sir John Lawrence... It makes all real business impossible... I keep the secret absolutely of where I am now & shall keep the secret (as long after my return as possible) of my return. And I shall make stringent rules (and I hope to keep them) after my return, as to only allowing messages to be brought me at certain hours – in order to set myself free for my real business - I take no "treatment" here, but old Mary (the bath woman whom Papa will remember at Umberslade) bathes me twice a day in the same way I do at home, which saves me much fatigue.' She said that she saw nothing but fog and snow except two mornings 'when I saw, I think, the most beautiful sunrises I ever saw in all my life – the clearest blue, the deepest violet, the most burning golden, the brightest red – over the whole valley. I always think that, except at Rome, there are no such sunrises as here'. She added 'I shall not come here again, tho' I consider that the absolute silence & solitude (except 10 minutes a day of Dr Johnson) has answered. For I mean, please God, quite certainly to come to my dearest mum this year. Ever your loving child, F'

Florence did visit Malvern once more. In January 1868 Benjamin Jowett wrote to Flo from Alfred Tennyson's house in Freshwater. 'I hope you will stay at Malvern as long as you possibly can. It was a happy thought going there...'

All that was wrong

The family was at the heart of much that was wrong in Florence's life. 'Why, Oh my God cannot I be satisfied with the life that satisfies so many people? What am I that their life is not good enough for me?' wrote she who preferred to listen to Faraday lecturing on electricity, or Sir Roderick Murchison on 'Scientifics', than sit sewing or gossiping.

In the nineteenth century, upper and middle-class women had their lives mapped out for them from the moment they were born. Their upbringing was devoted to making them marriageable and being a credit to their parents and husband. They were expected to dress fashionably, to be adept at needlework, drawing, music and painting. They should be able to write letters, make and receive social calls, make small talk, do charity work among the poor, and to be available at all times to do the bidding of parent or partner. This unfulfilling, useless waste of precious time was summed up by Florence's friend Mary Clarke as 'faddling, twaddling and the endless tweedling of nosegays in jugs'. Finding something more to her liking, in 1840 Florence began to study mathematics in the morning, getting up at 6am so that she would still have time to do her daily household duties afterwards. Her mother refused to let her have lessons. She hoped her daughter would get married, so learning mathematics would be a waste of time. For Flo, a necessary and fulfilling trade, occupation or profession was essential. 'I craved for some regular occupation, for something worth doing instead of frittering time away on useless trifles,' she wrote, but knew that there would always be opposition and difficulties.

In 1842, while she was at Lea Hurst, Florence visited the sick poor in their cottages in the nearby village of Holloway. In August 1845 her grandmother and her old nurse were ill and she nursed them both. With this experience came the knowledge and realisation of the importance that nurses should undergo a course of disciplined training, rather than assuming that all women were natural nurses. Eventually she asked her mother if she could go to Salisbury Infirmary for three months' training. Her mother was furious, and accused Florence of wanting to disgrace herself; Parthe became hysterical; her confused father left for London, wondering why such an education had been wasted on his younger daughter. Florence wrote to Hilary Bonham Carter, 'I shall never do anything and am worse than dust and nothing...' 'My misery and vacuity were indescribable.... I felt as if my soul would pass away in tears, in utter loneliness in a bitter passion of tears and agony of solitude....I cannot live, - forgive me, oh Lord, and let me die, this day let me die.'

Salvation appeared in the 1840s when, at Lord Ashley's suggestion, Florence started to get up early and study reports on the medical and sanitary conditions in hospitals throughout Europe. Each morning she made pages and pages of notes, but then came the breakfast bell. After breakfast she and Parthe were condemned to sit in the library with their father who read extracts from the newspaper to them. It was 'boring to desperation', she recalled. 'The most miserable exercise of the human intellect.' She said it was like lying on your back with your hands tied while someone poured liquid down your throat, except that if that happened you would suffocate, which would put an end to the misery. It was, to her, both a waste of her intellect and her time. 'In this cold and oppressive conventional atmosphere they* have never been satisfied in woman. But there was no point in complaining.' If anyone complained, those who did not suffer from the same feelings of repression would have as much understanding as a 'lizard would comprehend the sufferings of a Shetland sheep'. In 1851 Florence wrote that she could not expect any sympathy or help from her parents and sister. 'I have so long craved their sympathy that I can hardly reconcile myself to this. I have so long struggled to make myself understood, been sore, cast down, insupportably fretted by not being understood...'

To Florence, time was the most valuable of all things. She said that if someone had been robbed of half a crown, the police would be called. If a patient sat chatting to a doctor for an hour he would lose an hour's income, and would complain. 'But women have no right, because it is "only their time".' Florence wanted and needed unencumbered thinking time, but middle-class women 'are never supposed to have any occupation of sufficient importance not to be interrupted.... They have accustomed themselves to consider intellectual occupation as a merely selfish amusement, which it is their "duty" to give up for every trifler more selfish than themselves.'

* passion, intellect and moral activity

In *Cassandra* she relates how at social and domestic events women were expected to drop a remark every two minutes or they would be accused of sulking. It was tiresome and meant that there was no time to pursue one's own thoughts because they were always thinking of something to say. Without a moment's peace to themselves all day women went to bed feeling quite demented. She observed that if a woman had a physical pain, everyone would jump to attention and the doctor would be summoned immediately, yet her state of mind was utterly ignored. The only place where a woman would have the time to think for more than two minutes at a stretch would be in a monastery where there were rules and training for thought, and every day several hours were set aside for thinking.

There were several ways that a woman could escape this overpowering hell of family life and domestic misery. One was 'An indomitable force of character', possessed by women such as Elizabeth Garret Anderson, Mary Ann Evans, Harriet Martineau, Elizabeth Fry, and Marie Curie. The alternatives were marriage or widowhood, or if poverty or ill-health forced them to take up an occupation. The problem with marriage was that a wife's role was to command the servants, attend to the smooth-running of the household, and oversee the health and moral upbringing of their children. Married women could never discuss politics, religion or social questions with their husband because they had learned nothing that could feed or stimulate conversation. 'They talk about who shall come to dinner, who is to live in this lodge and who in that, about the improvement of the place or when they shall go to London.' Married women, she had heard, sometimes wished they could break a leg, or say they had got an infection, just to get a bit of time to themselves. Marriage was not for her. Having turned down offers of marriage from her cousin Henry Nicholson in 1845, and Richard Monckton Milnes, 'the man I adored', in 1849, she could say with certainty that, 'Some few [women] sacrifice marriage, because they must sacrifice all other life if they accept that.... A woman dedicates herself to the vocation of her husband.' 'Ladies work has always to be fitted in; where a man is, his business is the law.'

The monastery of ill-health

Florence would never be a widow, and never be poor, so ill-health was her only escape. On 1st November 1857 she and Aunt Mai, recently returned from Malvern, took a suite of rooms at the Burlington Hotel. Florence was still unwell so it was decided that she should be isolated from one of the chief causes of her illness – stress. Her retinue was reduced to three: Aunt Mai; Logan, a former surgical nurse who became her general handyman, and Clough, who visited twice daily to act as her secretary. Visitors were allowed by appointment only. Once, when Parthe offered to call on her, Florence replied: 'Dearie, It is very good of you to offer to come tomorrow but I could not see anyone, not if it were to save my life. I thought that you knew that I worked every day from 7:30 to 5:30 and that before 1:00 I could not see anyone except to save the Indian Empire.'

It is said that Florence lied to her mother and sister about her health and pretended to be ill to protect herself from their intrusion. However other visitors without appointments were also turned away, including General Gordon, Sophia, Queen of the Netherlands, and William Gladstone. Florence Nightingale was a prolific writer. Writers need to think; to organise notes, to draft and redraft; to make additions in the light of new information; to reach deadlines. Writing requires uninterrupted hours of work. With constant interruptions how could she have produced such a mass of published (and unpublished) work including *Notes on Matters Affecting the Health, Efficiency and Hospital Administration of the British Army* (1857), *Subsidiary Notes as to the Introduction of Female Nursing into Military Hospitals in Peace and War* (1858), *Suggestions for Thought* (1858-60), *Notes on Hospitals* (1859); *Notes on Nursing* (1860), *Observations of Disease in the Indian Army* (1862), *How People May Live and Not Die in India* (1863) and *Introductory Notes on Lying-in Institutions* (1871)?

As she wrote in *Cassandra* in 1852, the only way for a woman to have the time to think, and to carry out the work for which she was put on this earth, was to be ill or to feign illness. She realised during her months in Malvern that when she was ill her wishes were

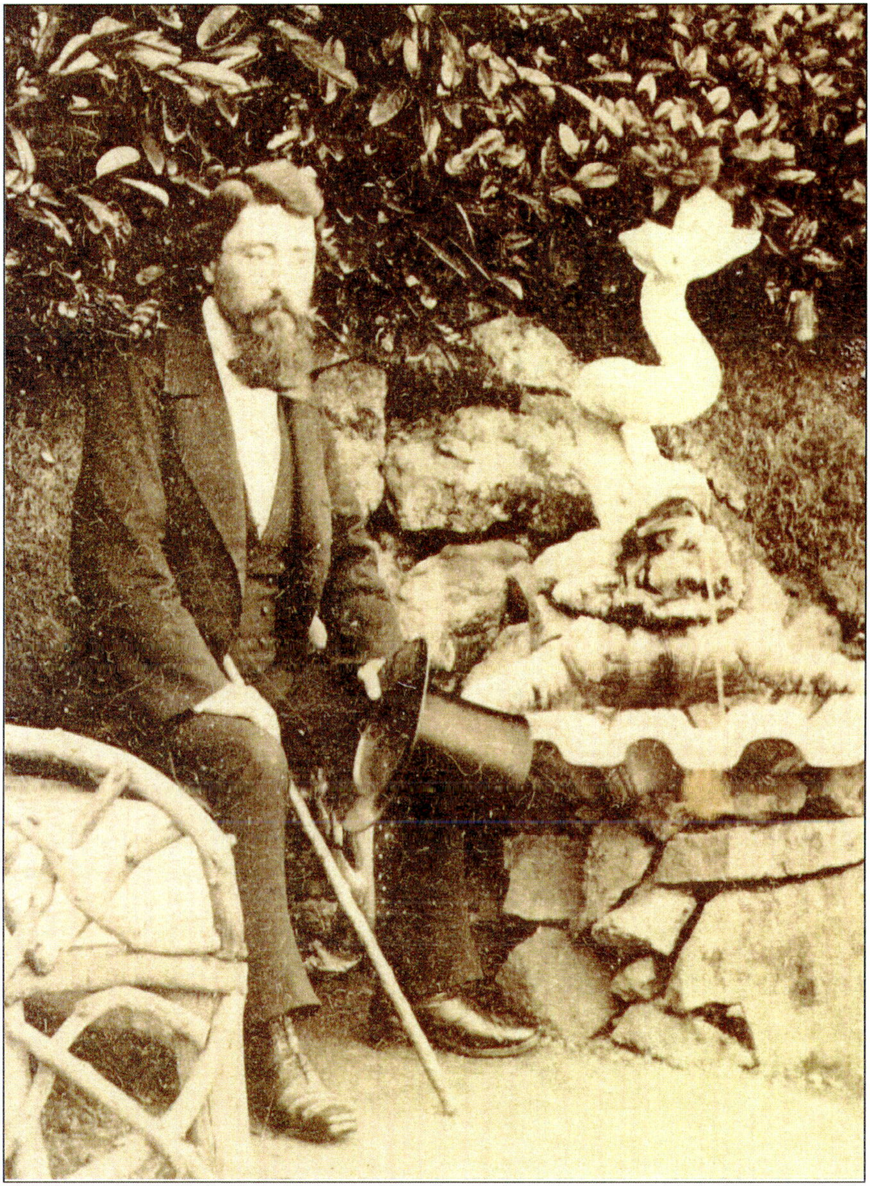

Dr Walter Johnson should be credited with doing more to save Florence Nightingale's life than any other man or woman. He is seen here seated by the drinking fountain at Malvernbury. Photograph courtesy of Brian Iles.

respected. Her strategy for survival and fulfilment was to take up a life where she rarely left her rooms. She gave up attending church and she gave up visiting her family. At last, for the first time in her life, she could concentrate on her work without the obstacles of interruption, constant unannounced visits, and unwanted demands from others. She ordered her life to eliminate stress, and instituted a bathing regime she had learned at Malvern that made her less fatigued. Knowing that where health is concerned prevention is better than cure, she became her own physician and psychiatrist who prescribed elective invalidism. There was no need to return to Malvern.

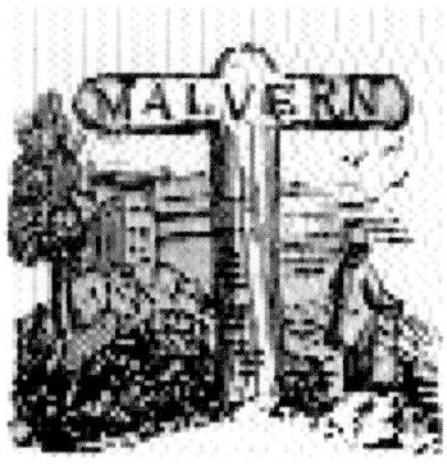

Bibliography

Anon, *Guide to Watering Places*, Longman, Rees, Orme and Green, London (1846)

Anon, *The Metropolis of the Water Cure by a restored invalid*, Simpkin, Marshall & Co, London (1858)

Bostridge, M., *Florence Nightingale: The Woman and Her Legend*, Viking (2008)

'Collected Works of Florence Nightingale' Vol 1, *Florence Nightingale: An Introduction to her Life and Family*, Lynn McDonald (ed.), Wilfrid Laurier University Press (2001)

'Collected Works of Florence Nightingale' Vol 7, *Florence Nightingale's European Travels*, Lynn McDonald (ed.), Wilfrid Laurier University Press (2004)

Cook, Sir Edward, *The Life of Florence Nightingale*, Macmillan & Co Ltd, London (Vol I 1820-1861; Vol II 1862-1910) (1913)

Cope, Zachary, *Florence Nightingale and the Doctors*, Museum Press Ltd (1958)

Florence Nightingale and the Crimea, 1854-55, official papers for the government enquiries into the first six months of the Crimean campaign, first published 1855 and 1856, reprinted by The Stationery Office (2000)

Gill, Gillian, *Nightingales: Florence and her Family*, Hodder and Stoughton Ltd (2004)

Granville, A.B., *The Spas of Germany*, Vols I & II, Brussels (1838)

Granville, A.B., *Spas of England: The Midlands and South* (first published 1841), Adams and Dart, Bath, Somerset (1971)

Groves, John, *Cowes, The Jewel of the Solent*, supported by the Rotary Club of Cowes (2002)

Gully, J.M., M.D, *The Water Cure in Chronic Disease*, John Churchill, London (1847)

Horn, Pamela (ed.), *Oxfordshire Country Life in the 1860s: The Early Diaries of George James Dew (1846-1928) of Lower Heyford*, Beacon Publications (1986)

Huxley, Elspeth, *Florence Nightingale*, Chancellor Press (1975)

Hunter, Adam M.D, *A Treatise on the Waters of Harrogate*, London (1846)

Lane, R., *Life at the Water Cure or A Month in Malvern*, Longman, Brown, Green, & Longmans, London (1846)

Lang, C.Y., and Shannon, E.F., (eds.), *The Letters of Alfred Lord Tennyson Volume I 1821-1850*,The Belknap Press of Harvard University Press (1981)
Metcalfe, R., *The Rise and Progress of Hydropathy in England and Scotland*, Simpkin, Marshall, Hamilton, Kent & Co Ltd, London (1906)
Nightingale, Florence, *Cassandra*, (1852) The Feminist Press, New York (1979)
Parsons, Charles, M.D, *Sea Air and Sea Bathing*, J & A Churchill, London (1877)
Pettinger, John W., *Tanworth in Arden*, Brewin Books (2005)
Quinn, E.V., & Priest, J.M (eds.), *Dear Miss Nightingale, a Selection of Benjamin Jowett's Letters 1860-1893*, Clarendon Press, Oxford (1987)
Small, Hugh, *Florence Nightingale, Avenging Angel*, Constable, London (1998)
Smedley, J., *Practical Hydropathy*, S.W Partridge, London (1861)
Soyer, A., *A Culinary Campaign*, (first edition 1857), Southover Press (1995)
Strachey, L., *Five Victorians*, The Reprint Society, London (1942)
Trail, R.T., M.D, *The Illustrated Hydropathic Encyclopaedia*, Fowler and Wells, New York (c.1870)
Turner, E.S., *Taking the Cure*, The Quality Book Club (1967)
Weaver, C., *Charles Darwin and Evelyn Waugh in Malvern*, Cora Weaver (2009)
Woodham Smith, Cecil, *Florence Nightingale*, (first edition 1950), Book Club Associates, London (1972)

Notes

WL - Wellcome Library, London (copies of originals held at Claydon House)
CHT - Claydon House Trust
BL ADD MSS - British Library, Additional Manuscripts
BWJ - Berrows Worcester Journal
F.N - Florence Nightingale
W.E.N - her father William Edward Nightingale
Fanny - her mother

Page

viii 'by the energy of...' quoted in Quinn, E.V & Priest, J.M (eds.), *Dear Miss Nightingale, a Selection of Benjamin Jowett's Letters 1860-1893*, p280
1 'I have no faith...' F.N to Mary Mohl (née Clarke), February 1851, quoted in Bostridge, M., *Florence Nightingale: The Woman and Her Legend,* p154
1 'I suppose you find...' quoted in the Catalogue of the Nightingale papers, CHT N15/23
4 'absence from...' F.N to Edwin Chadwick, 1860, BL ADD MSS 45,770 fl 71
5 'The first dip...' F.N to Fanny 19th October 1833, WL 8991/65 One of the main principles of hydropathy is that bathing in cold water warms the body, whereas bathing in hot water cools the body.
6 'a delightful summer...' Granville, A.B., *Spas of England: The Midlands and South*, p540
6 'Hot plunging...' Groves, John, *Cowes, The Jewel of the Solent*, p34
7 'Mrs Fowler...' BL ADD MSS 46,176 fl.28
7 'we drove through...' F.N to Parthe 6th October 1848 , WL 8993/1
8 'This morning the operation...' F.N to Parthe, 7th October 1848, WL 8993/2
9 'wicked old church', WL 8993/1
11 'I & the little birds...' F.N to W.E.N, 18th October 1848, WL 8993/3
13 'My treatment ...' F.N to Parthe, 22nd October 1848, WL 8993/4
14 'heaven knows how...' F.N to W.E.N, 18th October 1848, WL 8993/3
14 'a poor little Estonian...' F.N to Parthe, 1848, WL 8993/19
14 'old relations..' F.N to Parthe, November 1848, WL 8993/7 The Ladies Proby were Charlotte (1788-1860) and Frances (1789-1855), the two elderly spinster daughters of John Joshua Proby, 1st Earl of Carysfort. After the death of her sister, the elderly Lady Charlotte came alone to Malvern at the end of August 1857 and stayed for two weeks at Aucott House along the Worcester Road near Link Top.
15 'Your friend...' quoted in 'Collected Works' Vol 7, Lynn McDonald (ed.), p678

15 'Cold weather?' F.N to Parthe, 9th November 1848, WL 8993/6
15 'I get up...' F.N to Embley, November 1848, WL 8993/17
15 'we are both...' F.N to Richard Monckton Milnes, 29th November 1848, quoted in 'Collected Works' Vol 7, p677
16 'a highly popular amusement...' quoted in Cope, Z., *Florence Nightingale and the Doctors,* p129
17 'at six...' Lane, R., *Life at the Water Cure or A Month in Malvern,* p29-30
18 'mild atmosphere...' Gully, J., *The Water Cure in Chronic Disease,* p467
19 'It was an anxious...' Lane, R., *op.cit.*, p99
20 'it takes off languor...' Gully., J., *op.cit.,* p486
21 'A cold dripping sheet...' Smedley, J., *Practical Hydropathy,* p52
21 'a cold foot bath...' Gully, J., *op.cit.,* p509
21 'At 12 o'clock...' quoted in Weaver, C., *Darwin and Evelyn Waugh in Malvern,* p2
22 'Alfred is also...' Edward Firzgerald to Bernard Barton, 11th November 1848, quoted in Lang C. Y. and Shannon, E.F. (eds.), *The Letters of Alfred Lord Tennyson Volume I 1821-1850*, p295
25 'where nature ...' Granville, A.B., *The Spas of Germany*, Vol II, p157
26 'In all female...' Hunter, Adam M.D., *A Treatise on the Waters of Harrogate* p141
27 'we packed up...' F.N to Fanny, May 1852, WL 8993/124
27 'We bundled out...' F.N to Fanny, May 1852, WL 8993/124
28 'We are quite satisfied...' F.N to Fanny, 5th May 1852, WL 8993/84
28 'and not before..' F.N to Fanny, 13th May 1852, WL 8993/86
28 'having paid all... ' F.N to Fanny, 13th May 1852, WL 8993/86
29 'Dear Papa...' F.N to W.E.N 1st December 1851, WL 8993/50
31 'Mrs Johnson...' and 'Poor Cassandra..' F.N to Hilary Bonham Carter, 8th January, WL 8993/70
31 'a miserable little weed.... 'F.N to Fanny, 6th January 1852, WL 8993/69
31 'I like Johnson....' F.N to Fanny, 6th January 1852, WL 8993/69
31 'I however...' F.N to Fanny 8th January 1852, WL 8993 /70
33 'the cows...' F.N to Fanny, 8th January 1852, WL 8993/70
33 'I continue...' F.N to Hilary Bonham Carter, 8th January 1852, WL 8993/70
34 'I have been...' Parthe to Fanny, 19th September [1852] from Birk Hall, CHT 23
34 'I am taking...' 11th November 1852, WL 8993/116
35 'very lavish...' W.E.N to Fanny, 8th January 1852 , WL 8993/71
35 'He is a good...' F.N to Fanny, January 1852, WL 8993/69
35 'private supply...' *Malvern Advertiser*, 8th April 1893
38 very watchful ', very thoughtful.', Hilary Bonham Carter to Fanny, 21st January 1858, CHA, N212
40 'Ni lire...' quoted in Woodham Smith, C., *Florence Nightingale*, p260

41 'There were very...' *Florence Nightingale and the Crimea, (*extracts from the official papers for the government enquiry into the problems during the first six months of the Crimean campaign, August 1854 - January 1855, (first published 1855), p175
41 'No one can...' quoted in Woodham Smith, C., *op.cit.*, p278
42 'Here we are... Aunt Mai from Dr Gully's Ladies' Establishment, CHT 276
42 'Miss Florence...'*BWJ* and *The Worcester Herald,* 14th March 1857. On Saturday 7th March Flo wrote to Parthe saying she was hoping to be back in town [London] by the following Monday or Tuesday, so the newspaper reports were late with the 'news'.
44 'Miss Florence...' *The Preston Guardian*, 21st March 1857
44 'This benevolent lady...' *The Worcester Herald,* 21st March 1857. Using the Retail Price Index £20 would be approximately £1500 in 2009.
45 'Mounting guard...' Fanny to W.E.N 1857, CHT 308
45 'When I have...' Fanny to W.E.N, 17th August 1857, CHT 308
45 'and she came down....' and 'dismally poorly...' Parthe to W.E.N, 17th August 1857, CHT 308
45 'It is a scene...' quoted in Woodham Smith, C., *op.cit.*, p288
46 'She took...' and 'George is just...' undated, CHT 308 Dr Edward Johnson had retired from his practice at Ellerslie but his son Walter was practising at The Bury.
46 'Dearest Mother...' F.N to Fanny, 25th August 1857, WL 8997/48
47 'Her days...' quoted in Woodham Smith, C., *op.cit.,* p302
47 'The accounts of...' quoted in Cook, E.T., *The Life of Florence Nightingale*, Vol I 1820-1861 pp371-2
49 'ordinary terms...' Pamela Horn (ed.), *Oxfordshire Country Life in the 1860s: The Early Diaries of George James Dew (1846-1928) of Lower Heyford,* p36
49 'Please don't gull...' quoted in Cook, E.T., *op.cit.*, p 368
50 'the everlasting report...' Soyer, A., *A Culinary Campaign*, p100
50 'of her imprudence...' *ibid.* p137
51 'I am sorry...' quoted in Huxley, Elspeth , *Florence Nightingale*, p168
52 'Oh my poor...' WL 9020/14
52 'haunted by thoughts...' quoted in Bostridge, M., *op.cit.,* p298-9
52 'The cannon...' Soyer, A., *op.cit.*, p136
52 'that her state...' quoted in Bostridge, M., *op.cit.*, p328
53 'we regret...' *The Worcester Herald*, 26th December 1857
53 'much the same...', Aunt Mai [to Fanny?] December 1857, CHT 212
53 'the anxious tenor...' undated [December 1857?] Aunt Mai to W.E.N and Fanny, CHT 212
55 'her much tried experience...' Aunt Mai to Fanny, undated, CHT N212
58 'You know...' Hilary Bonham Carter to Fanny, 4th January 1858, CHT N212
58 'the work...' Hilary Bonham Carter to Aunt Mai, Tuesday 20th January 1858, CHT N212

58 'To my dearest Mother...' F.N to Fanny, 6th January 1858, WL 8997/60
60 'to rescue...' F.N to Fanny, 6th January 1858, WL 8997/60
61 'least excitement...' W.E.N to Fanny, 28th January 1858, CHT N70
62 'a most precarious state.' *Liverpool Mercury*, 2nd June 1859
62 'We regret to learn...' *The Derby Mercury*, 22nd February 1860; *Liverpool Mercury*, 17th February 1860
62 'MISS NIGHTINGALE'S HEALTH...' *BWJ*, 19th January 1861
62 'ILLNESS OF FLORENCE...' *The Penny Illustrated Paper*, 23rd November 1861
62 'very much worse...' Aunt Mai to Fanny, August 1861, CHT 89
64 'I should not...' F.N to Edwin Chadwick, 16th September 1860, BL ADD MSS 45,770 fl 178
64 'don't disparage...' F N to Edwin Chadwick, September 1860, BL ADD MSS 45,770 fl 183
65 'broke up...' quoted in Woodham Smith, C., *op.cit.*, p458
65 'As for my coming here...' F.N to Fanny, 11th January 1867, WL 9002/97
66 'I hope you...' quoted in Quinn E.V., & Priest, J.M., *op.cit.*, p. Jowett knew Malvern very well; he spent much time in West Malvern.
66 'Why, Oh my God...' Nightingale, F., *Cassandra*, p8
67 'faddling, twaddling...' quoted in Woodham Smith, C., *op.cit*, p35
67 'I craved for some...'quoted in Woodham Smith, C., *op.cit.*, p13
67 'I shall never do anything...' F.N to to Hilary Bonham Carter, 1841, quoted in Woodham Smith, C., *op.cit*, p40
67 'My misery and vacuity...' quoted in Woodham Smith, C., *op.cit.*, p60
68 'boring to desperation.' quoted in Woodham Smith, C., *op.cit.*, p60
68 'The most miserable...' F.N to to Hilary Bonham Carter, 1841, *ibid.*, p40
68 'a lizard...' Nightingale, F., *op.cit.*, p29
68 'I have so long...' quoted in Bostridge, M., *op.cit.*, p154
68 'But women...' Nightingale, F., *op.cit.*, p35
68 'are never supposed...' *ibid.,* p32
69 'An indomitable force of character', *ibid.*, p33
69 'They talk about..' *ibid.*, p44
69 'the man I adored', quoted in Woodham Smith, C., *op.cit.*, p76
69 'Some few women...' Nightingale, F., *op.cit.*, p40
69 'Ladies work...' Letter to to Hilary Bonham Carter, 1841, quoted in Woodham Smith, C., *op.cit.*, p40
70 'Dearie, It is very good of you...', F.N to Parthe c.1866-7 quoted in 'Collected Works' Vol I, p336

Index